ANATOMY OF FITNESS 501

High Intensity Interval Exercises

hinkler

Published by Hinkler Books Pty Ltd 2018, 2019
45–55 Fairchild Street
Heatherton Victoria 3202 Australia
www.hinkler.com

hinkler

© Hinkler Books Pty Ltd 2018
Created by Moseley Road Inc.
Cover Designer: Sam Grimmer
Prepress: Splitting Image
Production Director: Adam Moore
Project Art and Editorial Director: Lisa Purcell
Photographer: Naila Ruechel
Author: Charlotte van Aussel

ISBN: 9781 4889 4086 6

Printed and bound in Canada

ANATOMY OF FITNESS

501

High Intensity Interval Exercises

Craft perfect workouts for your own training goals
and discover the amazing hidden structure of your body

Contents

Chapter Two—Power Exercises 92

Introduction

Interval training helps you to maximize your workout efforts, whether at the gym, at home, or outdoors. This kind of training provides an effective cardio session that can also transform your physique with a variety of exercise types. It involves alternating intense bursts of movement with slowed-down recovery segments.

Gym-goers these days are increasingly turning to high-intensity regimens, whether they are signing up for tried-and-true aerobic and spin classes or checking out fitness boot camps, functional training programs, group dance classes, battle rope regimens, suspension training, cardio boxing workouts, or scores of other demanding disciplines. You can incorporate aspects of all of these—and more—to craft your own high-intensity interval training plan—a plan that will allow you to reap the greatest benefits for your hard work.

What is a high-intensity interval training program?

High-intensity interval training (HIIT) programs feature multiple components: classic cardio training, such as running and cardio machine work; functional fitness moves, like Mountain Climbers and Squats that use everyday movement patterns; and exercises like the Push-Up (and its scores of variations) that help you build power and strength. In these pages, you will find 501 of the best exercises to help you attain these benefits. You can incorporate them into a workout routine, add them to a strength-training regimen, or weave them into your cardio program. You can take the list to the gym, or you can perform most of them right at home or in your backyard.

This popular form of exercise combines two of the most effective fat-burning methods: a high-intensity component (like aerobic Mountain Climbers) and lower-intensity components (like strength-training Barbell Rows). The high-intensity component means that,

in a quick burst, you push your body to the absolute maximum in order to achieve muscle fatigue and maximum oxygen (keep in mind that the harder you work your muscles, the more oxygen they will require). Working your body at near-maximum levels triggers what is known as the afterburn effect—in other words, your body continues to consume oxygen and burn calories up to 48 hours after your workout. Of course, even elite athletes can only work at maximum levels for short bursts, so you need to incorporate intervals of lower-intensity activity. For example, you would first perform a five-minute warm-up like jumping rope, then follow that with an eight-rep set of a strength exercise like Barbell Rows, and then follow that with a one-minute burst of fast Mountain Climbers. You would then repeat the entire routine for a 45-minute session. Vary this type of training by alternating one of the many strength moves found in this book with any one of its cardio or plyometric moves or with cardio machine work.

Crafting your own workouts

There are probably just as many ways to put a workout program together as there are exercises to incorporate into it. Still, here are a few guidelines to help you figure out how to achieve your individual fitness goals. You can start by trying out a sampling of some of the featured exercises. Say that you want to work on lower-body toning—look for exercises like the many Squat

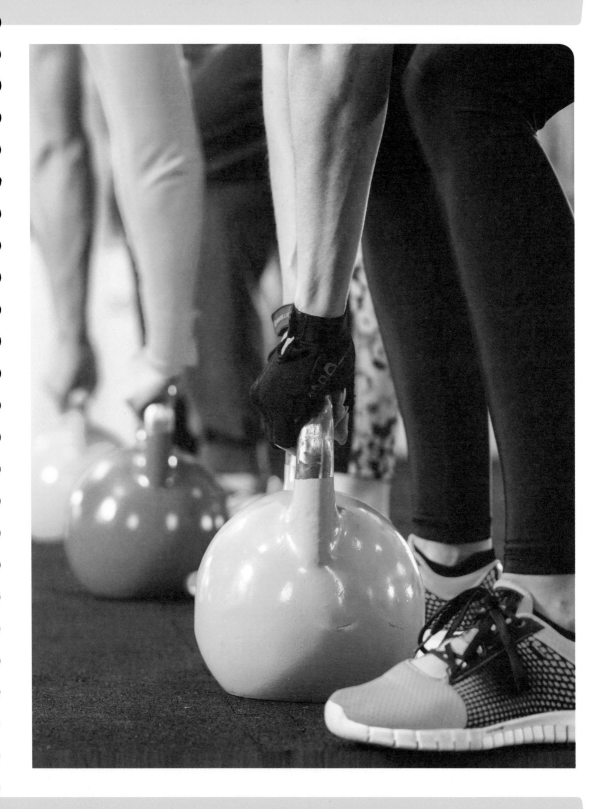

and Lunge variations. Want to burn fat? Try one of the jumps or some of the exercises labeled "plyo" or "plyometric," which are moves designed to incinerate calories and get your rate going. There are plenty, like the Burpees, that have multiple benefits, combining hard-core strength training with high-energy cardio.

Add in some classic cardio

Along with the exercises featured in the following pages, a well-rounded HIIT program includes classic cardio work—those rows and rows of exercise machines that fill just about every gym and health club these days. Most of them feature a setting for interval training so you don't even have to think about configuring your session. Here is a breakdown of a few of the most common cardio machines.

Treadmill The mainstay of both commercial gyms and home fitness rooms, a treadmill allows you to get in your daily run or walk no matter what the weather. Jogging at a moderate pace for a half hour will burn about 350 calories (1460 kJ). You can use it to walk, jog, or run on an even surface, or you can adjust the incline for a rigorous uphill workout. It helps you lose weight, tone muscle, relieve stress, and improve your cardiovascular health. For HIIT, if your treadmill has an "Interval" setting, activate it. While you are running, you can augment the lower-body emphasis with some upper-body work, such as throwing some punches. Try holding your arms close to your body, bent at about 90 degrees, and then jab outward with rotation, so that at the end of the motion your knuckles face away from your body. Alternate hands with a steady rhythm. You can also mix up your movements with side shuffles by setting the speed for two to four miles per hour (3.2 to 6.4 km), and pivoting to the side, holding on to

one of the treadmill handles for support, then shuffling sideways as the tread moves along. You can even try a backpedal by facing away from the console (making sure to keep a firm grasp on the handles) and walking or running backward.

Stationary bike This old-school piece of equipment offers high value. Working at a moderate pace, you can burn up to 650 calories (2720 kJ) per hour and improve heart and lung health, tone and strengthen muscles, and improve balance and coordination. It is also a low-impact form of exercise. You can find various versions at the gym—the standard upright, spin models, and recumbent styles that give you back support. To include this machine in a HIIT regimen, assume a "spinning" position—butt off the seat, arms braced on the handles, and weight forward. You can also amp up the resistance by adding weights. To do this, find a comfortable position, grab a dumbbell in each hand, and perform two sets curls or lateral raises.

Elliptical trainer No longer the new kid on the block, the elliptical trainer has become one of the most popular cardio machines: the go-to piece of equipment if you want an effective cardio workout with little stress on the joints. Spending a half hour on an elliptical will burn through 350 calories (1460 kJ). It can help with blood pressure, improve heart and lung health, and build stronger bones. To incorporate it into HIIT, it's as easy as adjusting the workout setting to "Interval" and following the routine through periods of high and low activity with varying levels of resistance for your desired time. To get the most benefit, halfway through your session change the direction to pedal backward.

Rowing machine Rowing machines are one of the cardio favorites of HIIT and functional training devotees, combining the best of a cardiovascular workout with powerful strength and endurance training. Rowing at a moderate pace for a half hour will burn about 200 calories (840 kJ) and improves heart and lung health, tones and strengthens muscles, helps you drop the pounds, and reduces stress.

Stair climber Also known as the stair machine, stair stepper, tread-climber or step machine, this star of the 1980s gym has proved its value over the years, becoming a favorite with gym-goers looking for a high-intensity workout. It offers efficient cardio, increases strength and body tone in your entire lower body, improves your balance, and engages your core muscles with every step. Working on a climber will burn

about 180 calories (750 kJ) in a half hour. You can also adjust the setting for "Interval," and try one of these variations—leg swings, double steps, or sidesteps, each for three to five minutes. To try the leg swing, swing your right leg behind you as you raise your left leg, and then keep alternating sides. For the double step, all you do is take two steps at a time. For the sidestep, stand sideways on the machine, making sure to securely hold on to the stability bar, and step up, placing one foot over the other. Midway through the interval, switch directions by pivoting 180 degrees and then continue by leading with the opposite foot.

Get to work!

Taken all together, combining a program of exercises and cardio will give you a high-intensity interval training workout. This kind of program will help you to build lean muscle, burn fat, improve heart health, and increase oxygen utilization, while you also improve your balance, posture, coordination, agility, endurance, flexibility, and power. The work may be hard, the sweat copious, but who wouldn't want these benefits?

Full-Body Anatomy

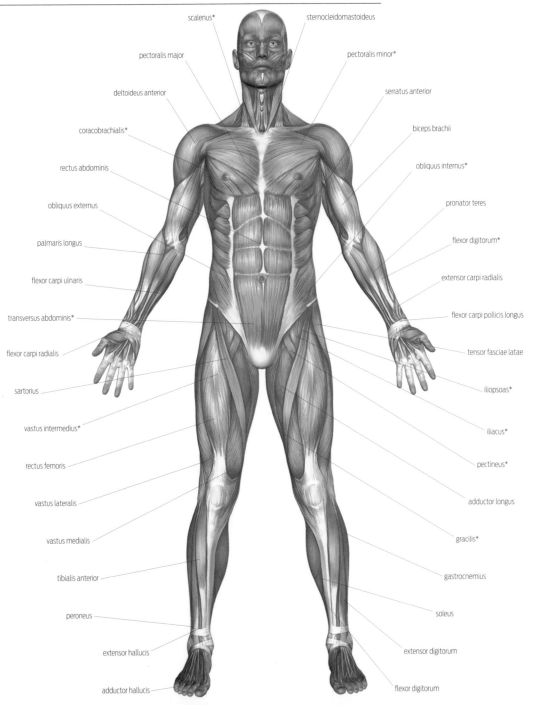

scalenus*

sternocleidomastoideus

pectoralis major

pectoralis minor*

deltoideus anterior

serratus anterior

coracobrachialis*

biceps brachii

rectus abdominis

obliquus internus*

obliquus externus

pronator teres

palmaris longus

flexor digitorum*

flexor carpi ulnaris

extensor carpi radialis

transversus abdominis*

flexor carpi pollicis longus

flexor carpi radialis

tensor fasciae latae

sartorius

iliopsoas*

vastus intermedius*

iliacus*

rectus femoris

pectineus*

vastus lateralis

adductor longus

vastus medialis

gracilis*

tibialis anterior

gastrocnemius

peroneus

soleus

extensor hallucis

extensor digitorum

adductor hallucis

flexor digitorum

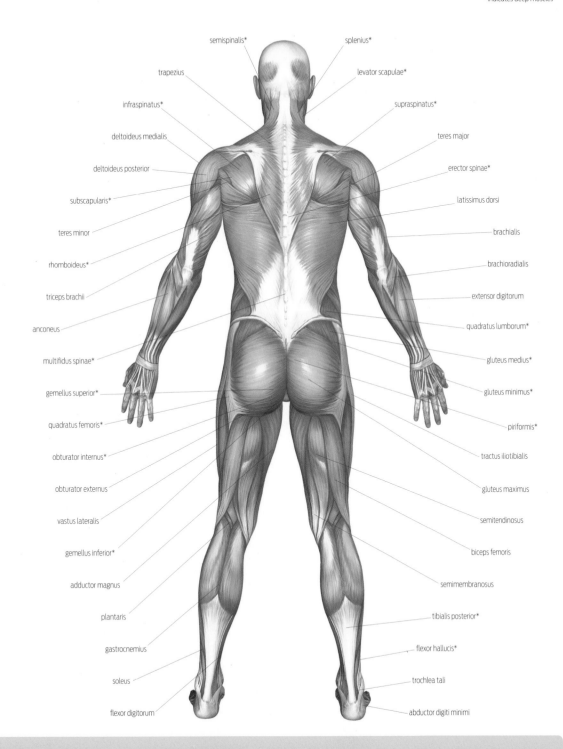

semispinalis*

splenius*

trapezius

levator scapulae*

infraspinatus*

supraspinatus*

deltoideus medialis

teres major

deltoideus posterior

erector spinae*

subscapularis*

latissimus dorsi

teres minor

brachialis

rhomboideus*

brachioradialis

triceps brachii

extensor digitorum

anconeus

quadratus lumborum*

multifidus spinae*

gluteus medius*

gemellus superior*

gluteus minimus*

quadratus femoris*

piriformis*

obturator internus*

tractus iliotibialis

obturator externus

gluteus maximus

vastus lateralis

semitendinosus

gemellus inferior*

biceps femoris

adductor magnus

semimembranosus

plantaris

tibialis posterior*

gastrocnemius

flexor hallucis*

soleus

trochlea tali

flexor digitorum

abductor digiti minimi

CHAPTER ONE

Functional Moves

In recent years, functional training has become an entrenched part of the fitness scene. This training method stresses real-life movement patterns like walking, running, pushing, pulling, carrying, hinging, squatting, and rotating. Building proficiency in these movement patterns can certainly enhance your everyday life, allowing you to perform common chores and activities with ease. Functional exercises also help you to attain the strength, stability, flexibility, and endurance needed for athletic pursuits. Revving up these kinds of exercises during high-intensity interval training boosts their aerobic benefits and also increases your power and builds muscle.

Functional Moves

001

Basic Squat

Often called the "king of all exercises," the squat—and its many variations—is a hard-working exercise that fits into just about any workout regimen, from concentrated bodybuilding to high-intensity boot camp training. It is a compound move that mimics natural, everyday movement patterns, working multiple joints and just about all your muscles, especially the thighs and glutes. Regularly performing squats can help you develop a strong core, increase lower-body strength and size, and promote joint health. Squats can also test your mental toughness; just try performing 20 well-executed reps.

rectus abdominis

vastus intermedius*

rectus femoris

sartorius

vastus medialis

gastrocnemius

adductor magnus

tibialis anterior

gluteus medius*

gluteus maximus

tensor fasciae latae

vastus lateralis

biceps femoris

soleus

- Stand with your legs and feet parallel and shoulder-width apart and your knees bent very slightly. Tuck your pelvis slightly forward, lift your chest, and press your shoulders down and back.

- Extend your arms straight out for stability, keeping them even with your shoulders. Plant your feet firmly on the floor, and curl your toes upward slightly.

- Draw in your abdominal muscles, and lower into a squat. Keep your heels planted on the floor and your chest as upright as possible, resisting the urge to bend too far forward. Exhale, and return to the original position. Repeat for the desired repetitions.

Correct form
A general rule of thumb is that you should only squat as low as you can while still maintaining a neutral, straight spine.

Avoid
Avoid sacrificing form for speed. The movement may look simple, but a poorly done squat can be hard on your hips, knees, and ankles.

002 Goblet Squat

Hold a dumbbell or kettlebell vertically next to your chest, with both hands cupping the dumbbell head or kettlebell handle, as if it were a heavy goblet. Keeping your abs braced, push your hips back and bend your knees to lower your body until your thighs are parallel to the floor. Pause, and then press upward back to the starting position, and repeat.

003 Sandbag Squat

Stand with your feet shoulder-width apart, holding a sandbag across your upper chest. Push your hips back and bend your knees to lower your body until your thighs are parallel to the floor. Drive your heels into the floor to explosively push yourself back up.

004 Resistance Band Squat

Secure a resistance band under both feet. Stand with feet shoulder-width apart, and then with an end in each hand, bring your hands to shoulder level. Keeping your knees aligned with your toes, bend your knees, and lower your body. Keeping your back straight, raise yourself back to the starting position, and repeat.

005 Squat and Row

Secure a resistance band to a sturdy object. Stand upright, holding both ends of the band. Plant your feet hip-width apart, making sure your back is neither arched nor slumped. In a smooth movement, begin to bend your knees. At the same time, bend your elbows as you pull both ends of the band in toward your body. Keeping the rest of your body stable and your abdominals engaged, use both hands to pull the band even further toward your body. Smoothly return to the starting position.

006 Press and Squat

Loop a resistance band around a weight machine. Stand facing away from the machine, your feet planted hip-distance apart or slightly wider. Grasp one handle in each hand and bend your elbows, feeling resistance from the band as you raise both handles to shoulder height. Bend your knees into a squat position as you straighten both arms in front of you, feeling resistance as you press. Gradually straighten your knees and draw your arms back, again bending your elbows to return to the starting position.

The Balance Ball Trainer

A balance ball trainer is an inflated rubber hemisphere attached to a rigid platform. You can use it with the dome side up or down. When facing up, the dome provides an unstable surface while the device itself remains stable. Facing down, it becomes highly unstable. Either side works to add functional balance challenges for athletic drills, aerobic activities, and other exercises.

007 Balance Ball Squat

Up the level of difficulty by performing a Basic Squat (#001) on the dome side of a balance ball.

008 Single-Leg Squat

Stand holding your arms straight out in front of your body at shoulder level. Raise your right leg, and cross it over your left so that your right ankle rests just above your left knee. Push your hips back, and lower your body as far as you can. Hold for a count of one, and then push your body back to the starting position.

009 Pistol Squat

Stand holding your arms straight out in front of your body at shoulder level. Raise your right leg off the floor, and hold it there. Push your hips back, and lower your body as far as you can. Hold for a count of one, and then push your body back to the starting position.

010 Dumbbell Squat

Grasp a dumbbell in each hand, and stand with your legs and feet parallel and shoulder-width apart. Keeping your knees aligned with your toes, bend your knees and lower your body into a squat position. Keeping your back straight, raise yourself back to the starting position, and repeat.

011 Power Squat

Stand straight, holding a weighted Medicine ball in front of your torso. Shift your weight to your left foot, and bend your right knee, lifting your right foot toward your buttocks. Bend your elbows, and draw the ball toward the outside of your right ear. Bend at your hips and knee, and lower your torso to the left, bringing the ball toward your right ankle. Press into your left leg and straighten your knee and torso, returning to the starting position, and repeat.

012 Barbell Squat

The Barbell Squat is the most commonly performed of the weighted squats. Also known as High Bar Back Squat or Olympic Squat, you hold the bar right at the base of your neck across the top of your trapezius muscles. There are many variations of a this kind of squat—it all depends on how and where you hold the barbell. In a Low Bar Barbell Squat, for example, the bar sits lower on your back, and in front versions, you hold it in front of your chest. No matter which version, the Barbell Squat is a key exercise for training your lower body. As with any exercise, form is essential, and safety is crucial—this kind of weight movement calls for a high level of mobility at the hips, spine, and shoulders.

· Set up the barbell on a squat rack so that it is at the same height as your upper chest. Position your body under the bar, with your knees bent so that the bar is resting high on the back of your shoulders.

· Grip the bar with your hands comfortably wider than your shoulders. Slowly straighten your legs to push upwards, lifting the barbell from the rack, and take one step forward.

· Standing with your legs shoulder-width apart, bend your knees forward and allow your hips to bend back as if you were sitting down until your thighs are parallel to the floor.

· Hold for a count of one, and then push up through your heels while straightening your hips and knees, until you have returned to the starting position. Repeat for the desired repetitions.

Correct form
Squeeze your butt to activate your glutes and hamstrings as you begin to rise from the squat.

Avoid
Avoid squatting straight down, which places too much stress on the knees. Instead, move as if you were sitting back into a chair so that you center your weight over your midfoot to heels.

013 Front Barbell Squat

Stand upright and take a barbell from a rack (or have a spotter help you), letting it rest along your upper chest. Position your feet shoulder-width apart with your toes pointed slightly outward. Move your shoulders back and your chest out so your back is flat and your torso erect. Cross your forearms in front of your chest so that your upper arms are parallel to the floor and each hand is grasping the bar near the opposite shoulder. Perform a Basic Squat (#001), and then push up through your heels while straightening your hips and knees to return to the starting position.

Suspension Training

Suspension cable systems, usually known as TRX (Total Resistance eXercise), are cropping up in gyms all over the world. TRX was developed by a former U.S. Navy SEAL using principles derived from rope training. In this form of body-weight resistance training, you perform a variety of multi-planar compound exercises, developing strength while using functional movements and dynamic positions. You can take advantage of your gym's set-up, but suspension systems are widely available for home use, too. The concept is an easy one—grab the cradles or hook your feet in them and then work your body against gravity. Performing suspension versions of traditional moves like squats, lunges, or push-ups adds an element of instability that helps you to build muscle and burn fat.

014 Suspended Squat

Use a TRX suspension system or loop a suspension band over a sturdy object. Face the anchor point of the band and grasp the band with both hands. Lower your hips down and back. Push up to return. Repeat for the desired repetitions.

015

Suspended Single-Leg Squat

Use a TRX suspension system or loop a suspension band over a sturdy object. Face the anchor point of the band and grasp the band with both hands. Stand on one leg, and lower your hips down and back. Push up to return. Repeat for the desired repetitions, and then switch sides.

Correct form

To perfect your form while training with suspension cables, start an exercise at the end range of the motion to find out how much tension you will need. This way you ensure that you have full tension throughout the whole movement.

Avoid

Avoid slacking. To obtain the full benefit of suspension training, resistance is crucial. If the straps aren't taut through the whole exercise, you aren't getting the necessary resistance.

016 Medicine Ball Squat
Grasping a weighted Medicine ball in both hands, stand with your legs and feet parallel and shoulder-width apart. Keeping your knees aligned with your toes, bend your knees, and lower your body into a squat position. Keeping your back straight, raise yourself back to the starting position, and repeat.

017 Chair Squat
Stand upright in front of a chair. Clasp your hands in front of your chest. Slowly lower into a squat position. Continue lowering until you are resting your butt on the chair. With control, rise back up to the starting position, and repeat.

018 Medicine Ball Chair Squat
Perform as you would the Chair Squat (#017), but challenge yourself by holding a Medicine ball in both hands at chest height in front of you throughout the exercise. This adds another level of resistance.

019 Box Squat with Side Leg Lift
Stand with your right foot on a step, grasping a disc weight or Medicine ball at waist level. Keeping your knees aligned with your toes, bend your knees and lower your body into a squat position. Keeping your back straight, raise yourself, shifting all your weight to your right foot as you lift your left leg straight out to the side. Return to the starting position, repeat for the desired repetitions, and then perform on the other leg.

020 Jump Squat
Place your fingers on the back of your head and pull your elbows back so that they're in line with your body. Dip your knees into a squat in preparation to leap, and then explosively jump as high as you can. When you land, immediately squat down, and jump again.

021 Resistance Band Jump Squat
Loop a resistance band over a sturdy object. Stand upright, holding both ends of the band in your hands. Your feet should be planted hip-width apart, your back neither arched nor slumped. Pull your arms back as you dip your knees into a squat in preparation to leap, and then explosively jump as high as you can. When you land, immediately squat down, and jump again.

022

Sumo Squat

Like any squat, the Sumo Squat is a terrific lower-body exercise that tones your thighs, butt, and calves. Its execution is similar to a Basic Squat, but your stance is wider and your toes are sharply angled away from the midline of your body. This kind of squat—which gets its name from the stance of a Japanese sumo wrestler—adds an inner-thigh focus to your workout. There are many variations, including weighted ones.

adductor longus
vastus lateralis

sartorius
pectineus*
rectus femoris
adductor brevis
vastus medialis
gracilis*
biceps femoris
obturator externus
obturator internus*
adductor magnus
soleus
gluteus maximus
gastrocnemius

Correct form
Imagine that you are balancing a book on top of your head. This will help you keep your chest elevated and the weight of your upper body over your hips.

Avoid
Avoid leaning your torso forward.

- Stand with your feet planted beyond shoulder width and your toes turned out. Bend your knees very slightly and tuck your pelvis slightly forward, lift your chest, and press your shoulders downward and back.

- Place your hands on your thighs.

- Squat down until your thighs are parallel to the floor, keeping your weight on your heels.

- Push off with your heels at the bottom of the squat, squeezing your glutes and inner thighs to rise back to the starting position.

023 Chair Plié

Stand with your feet in a wide stance with toes turned out and a chair in front of you. Keeping your knees aligned with your toes, bend your knees and lower your body into a squat position. Keeping your back straight, raise yourself back to the starting position, and repeat.

024 Side-Leaning Sumo Squat

Begin at the bottom position of a Sumo Squat (#022), with your knees bent and thighs parallel to the floor. Drop your right forearm onto your right thigh, just above the kneecap. Bring your left arm and hand straight up and reach over to the right side. Hold this position as you stretch. Round your left arm down so that both forearms are on your thighs, and bring your head back to the center. Push off with your heels at the bottom of the squat, squeezing your glutes and inner thighs to rise back to the starting position. Switch sides, and repeat, alternating right and left reaches.

025 Toe-Touch Sumo Squat

Perform as you would a Sumo Squat (#022), and then bend forward to touch your toes. Return to standing position, and repeat.

026 Toe-Touch Sumo Squat with Reach

Perform as you would a Toe-Touch Sumo Squat (#025), and then at the bottom of the move, rotate your torso to extend one arm toward the ceiling. Return to the toe-touch position, and then extend the opposite arm. Return to standing position, and continue, alternating toe touches and arm reaches.

027 Medicine Ball Sumo Squat with Overhead Lift

Stand holding a Medicine ball at chest height. Perform as you would a Sumo Squat (#022), extending your arms straight downward. As you return to standing position, lift the ball straight up toward the ceiling. Continue lowering and raising the ball as you alternate squatting and standing.

028 Weighted Sumo Squat

Stand holding a weight such as a disc weight, kettlebell, dumbbell, or Medicine ball, and perform as you would a Sumo Squat (#022).

029

Split Squat

The Split Squat uses a staggered stance, with one foot placed forward of the other. This move is often confused with a lunge—the key difference between the two is your rear leg. In a split squat, you do not move your rear foot throughout the entire exercise. In a lunge, you engage your rear leg, using both legs at the same time. Like a regular squat, a split squat works your lower body, but places greater emphasis on the hamstrings, gluteus medius, and external obliques. Your back also remains more erect in a properly executed split squat.

iliopsoas*

rectus femoris

vastus lateralis

vastus intermedius*

vastus medialis

gastrocnemius

sartorius

soleus

Correct form
Point your knees in the same direction as your feet throughout the movement, and keep your torso upright as you lower into the squat.

Avoid
Avoid extending your leading knee past your toes.

Annotation Key
Bold text indicates target muscles
Black text indicates other working muscles
* indicates deep muscles

gluteus medius*

gluteus maximus

semitendinosus

biceps femoris

semimembranosus

- Stand with your arms at your sides or with your hands on your hips. Position your feet far apart: one foot forward and the other foot behind.

- Squat down by bending your front leg. Allow the heel of your rear foot to rise up while the knee of your rear leg bends slightly until it almost makes contact with the floor. Return to the original standing position by straightening your forward leg. Repeat for the desired repetitions and then switch sides.

030 Dumbbell Split Squat

Hold a pair of dumbbells in each hand, letting them hang at arm's length at your sides, your palms facing each other. Perform a Split Squat (#029), pause, and then push yourself back up to the starting position as quickly as you can. Switch legs, and repeat, continuing to alternate sides for the desired repetitions.

031 Split Squat with Band Row

Stand in a staggered stance, holding both ends of a resistance band (or suspension cables) in your hands. Bend one leg behind you to form a split squat while holding the band taut. At the same time, bend your elbows as you pull the band in toward your body. Keeping the rest of your body stable and your abdominal muscles fully engaged, use both hands to pull the band even closer to your body. Smoothly return to the starting position, and repeat for the desired repetitions. Switch sides, and perform with the other leg behind.

032 Split Squat with Band Curl

Holding both ends of a resistance band, perform a Split Squat (#029) while holding the band taut. At the same time, bend your elbows as you pull both ends of the band in toward your body. Keeping the rest of your body stable and your abdominal muscles engaged, use both hands to pull the band even closer to your body. Smoothly return to the starting position, and repeat for the desired repetitions. Switch sides and perform with the other leg behind.

033 Medicine Ball Split Squat

Perform as you would a Split Squat (#029) while holding a Medicine ball with both hands at arm's length in front of you. Raise the ball to shoulder height as you descend, and bring it back down as you rise back up.

034 Overhead Sandbag Split Squat

Stand in a staggered stance, holding a sandbag with both hands at arm's length in front of you. Bend both knees into a split squat position as you simultaneously extend your arms over your head so that the sandbag flips behind you. Smoothly return to the starting position, and repeat for the desired repetitions. Switch sides and perform with the other leg behind.

035 Bulgarian Split Squat

Also known as the Rear-Foot-Elevated Split Squat, the Bulgarian Split Squat calls for you to elevate your back non-moving leg. This squat variation can be an antidote to the effects of too much time spent in front of a computer—sitting for long periods can cause the hip flexor and quadriceps muscles to shorten. The Bulgarian Split Squat counteracts that by helping you to increase the strength and flexibility of your hip flexors and quadriceps while not placing too much stress on your lower back.

· Stand in a staggered stance with your right leg behind you and the ball of your foot resting on an elevated surface, such as an aerobic step or weight bench. You can hold a weight such as a disc weight or Medicine ball, or use just your body weight.

· Bend both knees into a split squat position.

· Smoothly return to the starting position, and repeat for the desired repetitions. Switch sides and perform with the other leg behind.

036 Swiss Ball Bulgarian Split Squat

Stand lunge-length in front of a Swiss ball. Rest the top of your right foot on the ball behind you. Lower your body until your front knee is bent at a 90-degree angle. Squeeze your thighs together to keep your balance. Switch legs, and perform on the other side.

037 Bulgarian Split Squat with Overhead Press

Stand in a staggered stance with your elbows bent to form right angles. Perform a Bulgarian Split Squat (#035) as you raise both arms to shoulder height. Smoothly return to the starting position, and repeat for the desired repetitions. Switch sides and perform on the other leg.

038 Bulgarian Split Squat with Dumbbell Overhead Press

Stand in a staggered stance holding a dumbbell in each hand. Perform a Bulgarian Split Squat (#035) as you extend the dumbbells over your head. Smoothly return to the starting position, and repeat for the desired repetitions. Switch sides and perform on the other leg.

039

Wall Sit and Squat

A variation of the classic squat, the Wall Sit is a great way for exercise newbies to perfect their squatting form before advancing on to the more difficult versions of the squat. Aim for five sets of minute-long sits: with practice, you will gain core, back, and leg strength and hip and knee mobility, allowing you to squat lower.

Annotation Key
Bold text indicates target muscles
Black text indicates other working muscles
* indicates deep muscles

rectus abdominis

obliquus externus

transversus abdominis*

rectus femoris

vastus intermedius

vastus lateralis

tibialis anterior

tensor fasciae latae

gluteus maximus

gastrocnemius

tibialis posterior*

extensor digitorum longus

flexor hallucis

extensor hallucis

Correct form
Keep your back straight.

Avoid
Do not allow your shoulders to round forward or your knees to come past your toes.

- Stand with your feet planted beyond shoulder width and your toes turned out. Bend your knees very slightly and tuck your pelvis slightly forward, lift your chest, and press your shoulders downward and back.

- Place your hands on your thighs.

- Squat down until your thighs are parallel to the floor, keeping your weight on your heels.

- Push off with your heels at the bottom of the squat, squeezing your glutes and inner thighs to rise back to the starting position.

040 Swiss Ball Wall Squat

Place a Swiss ball against a wall and stand so that your back and shoulders are pinning it to the wall. Your feet should be about hip-width apart, but slightly ahead of your hips. Raise your arms straight out in front of you so that they are parallel to your thighs, and relax your upper torso. Keeping the ball pinned against the wall, slowly bend your hips and knees as you lower to a sitting position, rolling the ball down the wall with you as you sit. Hold for a count of 10, and then press back to the starting position, rolling the ball up the wall with your shoulders as you rise.

041 Swiss Ball Squat with Biceps Curl

Stand at a wall with the Swiss ball against your back, grasping a dumbbell in each hand. Plant your feet slightly in front of your torso to prepare. Bend your knees and lower toward the floor while curling the dumbbells toward your chest. As you lower into the squat position, keep the Swiss ball securely behind your back. Gradually straighten your arms and legs as you rise to stand and release the dumbbells to your sides.

042 Single-Leg Swiss Ball Squat with Biceps Curl

Perform as you would a Swiss Ball Squat with Biceps Curl (#041), but while in the squatting and curling position, extend one leg, hold, and then release. Repeat on the other side.

Choosing the Right Swiss Ball

A Swiss ball (also called a fitness ball, exercise ball, gym ball, physioball, and many other names) is a flexible, inflatable PVC ball with a host of fitness uses, including balance training, physical therapy, and many kinds of strength and cardio exercises. It is available in many sizes, from approximately 14 to 34 inches (36 to 86 cm) in circumference. If you want to get the most out of this piece of equipment, you must work with a ball of the correct size for your height. Exact sizes can vary from manufacturer to manufacturer, but this chart will give you a general guide to choosing the right size. Many come with their own pump—make sure to fill yours until it is firm, but still with a bit of give.

YOUR HEIGHT	BALL SIZE	BALL HEIGHT
Up to 4 feet 7 inches (140 cm)	Extra Small	14 inches (36 cm)
4 feet 7 inches to 5 feet (140 to 152 cm)	Small	18 inches (46 cm)
5 feet to 5 feet 6 inches (152 to 168 cm)	Medium	22 inches (56 cm)
5 feet 6 inches to 6 feet 1 inch (168 to 185 cm)	Large	26 inches (66 cm)
6 feet 1 inch to 6 feet 8 inches (185 to 203 cm)	X Large	30 inches (76 cm)
Over 6 feet 8 inches (203 cm)	XX Large	34 inches (86 cm)

043

Forward Lunge

The lunge is an important group of exercises that strengthen your lower body. There are many variations, but all will efficiently work your glutes, quadriceps, and hamstrings—and regularly engaging these large muscle groups can speed up your metabolism. Begin with the familiar Forward Lunge—a highly functional exercise that closely mimics your walking pattern while challenging your balance.

Annotation Key
Bold text indicates target muscles
Black text indicates other working muscles
* indicates deep muscles

iliopsoas*
adductor brevis
pectineus*
adductor longus
gluteus minimus*
vastus medialis
gluteus maximus
gracilis*
biceps femoris
semitendinosus
tensor fasciae latae
vastus intermedius*
semimembranosus
vastus lateralis
rectus femoris
adductor magnus

Correct form
Engage your core when executing a lunge. To control the tilt of your pelvis as you flex one hip and extend the other, your hip, abdominal, and lower-back muscles must work synergistically.

Avoid
Don't look down. To help you maintain a straight upper body, relax your shoulders, and keep your chin up, gazing at a point in front of you. This will help you avoid rounding your neck and upper back.

· Stand with your legs and feet parallel and shoulder-width apart, your knees bent very slightly. Tuck your pelvis slightly forward, lift your chest, and press your shoulders down and back.

· Take a big step forward with your right leg, and start to shift your weight forward so that your heel hits the floor first.

· Lower your body until your right thigh is parallel to the floor and your right shin is vertical. Lightly tap your left knee to the floor while keeping your weight on your right heel.

· Press into your right heel to drive back up to the starting position. Switch legs, and repeat on the other side.

044 Forward Lunge with Twist

Perform as you would a Forward Lunge (#043), but at the bottom of the movement, place your hands on the floor on the inside of your right foot, and then guide your right arm up toward the ceiling, twisting your torso. Return to the center, and repeat on the other side.

045 Straight-Leg Lunge

Stand with your legs and feet parallel and shoulder-width apart. Bend your knees very slightly and tuck your pelvis slightly forwards, lift your chest, and press your shoulders downward and back. Keeping both legs straight, take a big step forward with your right leg, and lean your torso forward over your right leg, placing your hands on your knee. Return to standing, and repeat on the other side.

046 Straight-Leg Lunge with Floor Touch

Perform as you would a Straight-Leg Lunge (#045), but rather than stopping at the knee, lean your torso forward as far as you are able, aiming to place your hands flat on the floor on either side of your front foot. Return to the starting position, and repeat on the other side.

047 Forward Lunge Pass Under

Stand with your feet together, holding a Medicine ball at chest height. Take a big step forward with your left foot, and lower into a lunge. Hinge at the waist as you shift the ball into your right hand, bringing it beneath your left thigh to pass it to your left hand. Return to the starting position, and then repeat on the other side.

048 Forward Lunge with Rear Leg Raise

Perform a Forward Lunge (#043) with your right leg forward. As you straighten your right leg, hinge forward at the hips and lift your straightened left leg off the floor behind you until it's about parallel to the floor. Return to the starting position, and then repeat on the other side.

049 Tick-Tock Lunge

Perform a Reverse Lunge (#059) with your right leg behind you. Push off your right foot, and immediately take a big step forward into a Forward Lunge (#043). Perform the desired reps, and then repeat the sequence, starting with your left leg.

050 Twisting Lunge

Stand with your feet shoulder-width apart and your arms extended at shoulder height, palms down. Perform a Forward Lunge (#043), twist your torso to the right, and reach your right hand back to touch your left heel while extending your left arm straight up. Return to the starting position, and repeat on the opposite side.

051 Diagonal Lunge

Perform as you would a Forward Lunge (#043), but instead of moving in a straight line, step out on a diagonal. Return to the starting position, and then repeat on the other side.

052 Diagonal Jumpers

Perform as you would a Forward Lunge (#043) with your right leg in front. Then, straighten both legs. Jump up to switch legs so that your left leg is in front. Take a moment to find your balance. Bend both knees to sink down into another lunge. Straighten your knees and then keep repeating for the desired repetitions.

053 Dumbbell Lunge

Stand up straight with a tight core, holding dumbbells at your sides, and perform as you would a Forward Lunge (#043).

054 Barbell Lunge

The Barbell Lunge is one of the most effective exercises for improving coordination and upping athleticism. Executed properly, it will help you to strengthen the muscles needed for many real-life movements like sprinting, jumping, and climbing stairs. When attempting this move, caution should be exercised as well as your muscles—it requires a great deal of balance. It is also safest to perform this lunge inside a squat rack.

- Stand holding a barbell across your shoulders with an overhand grip, and your feet about shoulder-width apart.

- Keeping your head up, back straight, and chest high, step one foot forward, bending your knees, and bring your back knee almost to the floor.

- Push yourself back up to the starting position with one strong, controlled thrust. Repeat the movement, stepping forward with the other foot.

Walking Lunge

Like the Forward Lunge, the Walking Lunge is a dynamic stretch that stabilizes your knees while building strength in your thigh muscles, both front and back. The Walking Lunge also efficiently works your glutes to firm and lift your butt, and the forward progression adds cardio intensity.

Correct form
Try to drop your back knee as close to the ground as you can without touching it. Bend your front knee so that it is directly over your ankle.

Avoid
Avoid leaning forward—keep your torso erect.

gluteus maximus

vastus intermedius*

iliopsoas*

rectus femoris

sartorius

vastus lateralis

gastrocnemius

vastus medialis

Annotation Key
Bold text indicates target muscles
Black text indicates other working muscles
* indicates deep muscles

gluteus medius*

semitendinosus

biceps femoris

semimembranosus

- Stand with your legs together and your arms hanging at your sides.

- Take a large step forward with your left leg.

- Lower your right knee to the floor, and then forcefully push off your left foot to return to standing position. Repeat on the other side, and continue to alternate your leading leg as you move forward for the desired steps.

056 Dumbbell Walking Lunge

Stand with your legs together and your arms at your sides, a dumbbell in each hand, and perform as you would a Walking Lunge (#055).

057 Reach-and-Twist Walking Lunge

Stand with feet about hip-width apart and your torso facing forward. Hold a weighted Medicine ball in both hands. Lunge your left foot forward. Begin to bend both knees, lowering your whole body into the lunge. At the same time, raise the Medicine ball until it is over your left shoulder. In a single motion, rise up to stand, bringing the ball back to center, and then perform the lunge and reach in the other direction. Continue to lunge and move the ball from side to side as you walk forward.

058 Jumping Lunge

The quick pace of this exercise intensifies the already hard-working lunge, demonstrating how the principles of plyometrics can add intensity to a basic exercise.

- Stand upright with your feet hip-width apart and your arms at your sides. With your right leg, take a big step forward.

- Bend both legs to lower into a deep lunge, and then straighten both legs.

- Lifting your arms overhead, jump up to switch legs so that your left leg is in front. Take a moment to find your balance when you land.

- Bend both knees to sink down into another lunge. Straighten your knees, and then keep repeating for the desired time or repetitions.

Up the Intensity with Plyometric Movements

Probably one of the easiest—and arguably one of the most efficient—ways to up the intensity of your interval workout regimen is to include plenty of plyometric moves. The plyometrics method, also known as jump training, calls for you to focus on quickly moving a muscle from extension to contraction in an explosive manner, such as in repeatedly alternating jumps and squats. Used by athletes and martial artists to improve performance, high-energy plyometric exercises can increase power, speed, and strength.

059

Reverse Lunge

Like the Forward Lunge, the Reverse Lunge is an excellent lower-body exercise. Also known as the Step-Back Lunge, this lunge variation offers your body a challenge by moving you backward—a direction you probably don't move in very often. Some proponents prefer this version over its opposite, because its backward momentum keeps your body in the optimal lunge position—your weight is on your heel with your knee above your ankle. This is a great exercise to prepare you for sports and other activities that require speed and power, particularly sprinting, but it is also the less difficult of the two basic lunges, and it is often a good option for anyone with a balance problem.

rectus abdominis

iliopsoas*

transversus abdominis*

vastus intermedius

sartorius

gluteus medius*

rectus femoris

gluteus maximus

vastus medialis

adductor longus

tensor fasciae latae

adductor magnus

soleus

flexor digitorum

vastus lateralis

gastrocnemius

gracilis

semitendinosus

biceps femoris

semimembranosus

- Stand with your hands on your hips and your feet shoulder-width apart.

- Take a big step backward, bending your knees as you do so.

- When your front thigh is roughly parallel to the floor, push through your front heel to return to the starting position.

- Switch legs, and repeat on the other side.

Correct form
To fully engage your glutes, press the heel of your front foot into the floor as you lift up.

Avoid
Avoid extending your front knee past your toes.

060

Dumbbell Reverse Lunge
To add resistance, perform a Reverse Lunge (#059) while holding a dumbbell in each hand.

061

Barbell Reverse Lunge
Holding a barbell across your shoulders with an overhand grip, perform a Reverse Lunge (#059). Press through your heel and glutes and explosively ascend back up to the starting position. Repeat a full set on one side, and then switch to the opposite side.

062

Kettlebell Overhead Reverse Lunge
Stand with your feet hip-width apart. Hold a kettlebell in your right hand and extend your left arm straight out to the side. Press the kettlebell overhead, then with the weight locked out directly above you, perform a Reverse Lunge (#059), lowering your left knee until it nearly touches the floor. Flex through your hips again to raise your torso back up to a standing position. Repeat with alternating legs and arms.

063

Lateral-Extension Reverse Lunge
Stand with your feet hip-width apart and your arms at your sides or on your hips. Perform a Reverse Lunge (#059) as you raise your arms to the side until they are level with your shoulders. Return to the starting position by extending the hip and knee of your left leg and bringing your right leg forward to meet your left. Repeat with alternating legs and arms.

064

Dumbbell Lateral-Extension Reverse Lunge
To add resistance, perform a Lateral-Extension Reverse Lunge (#063) while holding a dumbbell in each hand.

065

Reverse Lunge with Chest Press
Stand with your feet hip-width apart. Loop a resistance band around a stable object and grasp a handle in each hand. Raise your arms to hold both bands perpendicular to your body, slightly taut. Step your left leg behind you. Perform a Reverse Lunge (#059), at the same time lowering both arms, feeling resistance in the bands. Gradually straighten your legs and raise your arms to your sides to return to the starting position. Step your left leg forward and repeat on the other side.

066 Reverse Lunge Knee-Up

Perform as you would a Reverse Lunge (#059), but instead of returning to standing position, in one explosive motion, straighten your front leg to jump up and draw your back leg up in front of you so that your thigh is parallel to the floor. Return to the Reverse Lunge stance and repeat for the desired repetitions. Repeat on the other side.

067 Reverse Lunge and Kick

Perform as you would a Reverse Lunge (#059), but instead of returning to a standing position, kick your back leg out in front of you until you can touch your toes with your opposite hand. Return to a standing position, and repeat on the other side.

068 Suspended Reverse Lunge

Loop a suspension band over a sturdy object. Standing in a staggered stance, face away from the anchor point and suspend your back foot through the looped band. Lower into a lunge, keeping your torso erect until both knees form 90-degree angles. Drive back up by pushing through your front heel.

069 Low Lunge

Stand with your feet hip-width apart. Bend your knees and step back with your right foot, keeping your legs in line with your hips. Press the ball of your right foot on the floor and contract your thigh muscles as you bring your hands to either side of your left foot. Return to a standing position and repeat on the opposite side.

070 Crescent Lunge

Perform a Low Lunge (#069), and at the bottom of the movement, drop your back knee to the floor. Bring your hands onto your front knee, making sure the knee is directly over your ankle. Inhale and raise your arms above your head, keeping your arms in line with your ears. Lower your arms, return to a standing position and then repeat on the opposite side.

071 Low Lunge with Reach

Perform a Low Lunge (#069), and at the bottom of the movement, bring your hands to the front knee. Inhale and reach forward with both arms. Return to the start and repeat with the other leg.

072

Lateral Lunge

The Lateral Lunge introduces a new plane of movement to lunge or squat exercises. Rather than a forward or backward motion, which takes place in the sagittal plane that divides the body into left and right, the side-to-side motion moves you in the frontal plane, which divides the body into back and front portions. A Lateral Lunge also calls for each leg to work independently, so your dominant leg cannot take on a greater share of the work. This kind of lunge has many variations that you can add to your workout regimen. Just perform as many reps as possible for one to two minutes on each side, or plug one of its variations into a high-intensity circuit.

Correct form
Keep your chest up, your shoulders down, and your upper arms parallel to the floor throughout the exercise. Be sure to engage your glutes as you lunge.

Avoid
Don't crane your neck as you perform the movement. Avoid lifting your feet off the floor.

deltoideus anterior
transversus abdominis*
vastus intermedius*
adductor magnus
sartorius
gracilis*

deltoideus medialis
obliquus externus
gluteus medius*
gluteus maximus
tensor fasciae latae
iliopsoas*
adductor longus
rectus femoris
biceps femoris
gastrocnemius
vastus medialis
vastus lateralis
soleus

Annotation Key
Bold text indicates target muscles
Black text indicates other working muscles
* indicates deep muscles

- Stand upright with your arms outstretched in front of you, parallel to the floor.

- Step out to the left. Squat down on your right leg, bending at your hips while maintaining a neutral spine. Begin to extend your left leg, keeping both feet flat on the floor.

- Bend your right knee until your thigh is parallel to the floor, and your left leg is fully extended.

- Keeping your arms parallel to the floor, squeeze your glutes and press off your right leg to return to the starting position and repeat. Perform the desired reps, then repeat on the other side.

073 Curtsy Lunge

Stand upright with your feet together and your arms outstretched in front of you, parallel to the floor. Take a big step back with your right leg, crossing it behind your left leg. Bend both knees, and lower your body until your front thigh is parallel with the floor. Return to the starting position, and repeat on the other side.

074 Clock Lunge

This exercise combines the three basic lunges into one. Stand with your legs and feet parallel and shoulder-width apart and your knees very slightly bent. Tuck your pelvis slightly forward, lift your chest, press your shoulders down and back, and then perform a Forward Lunge (#043). Return to standing position, and then perform a Lateral Lunge (#072). Return to standing position, and then perform a Reverse Lunge (#059). Return to a standing position, and repeat in the opposite direction.

075 Lateral-Extension Lateral Lunge

Stand with your feet hip-width apart and your arms at your sides, a dumbbell or hand weight in each hand. Take a big step to the left, performing a Lateral Lunge (#072). At the same time, raise both arms so they are parallel to the floor, forming a straight line. Smoothly and with control, return to the starting position. Repeat on the other side.

076 Side Lunge Stretch

From the Sumo Squat (#022), drop your hands onto the floor in front of you, transferring some of your weight onto your arms. Staying as low as possible, shift your body over to the right, bending your right knee and extending and straightening your left leg. Return to the center, switch sides, and repeat.

077 Single-Leg Lateral Lunge with Lift

Grasp a dumbbell in each hand with palms facing each other. Perform a Lateral Lunge (#072) on your left leg as you lean your torso slightly forward until the weights are at knee level. As you straighten your left leg, lift your right leg out to the side until it is almost parallel to the floor. Lower your right leg back to the lateral lunge, and then return to standing. Repeat on the other side.

078 Alternating Touchdown Lunge

Perform a Lateral Lunge (#072) to the right, keeping your back straight and chest high as you bring your left arm across your body to touch your right toes. Reverse the movement, and return to standing position. Repeat on the other side and continue alternating sides.

079 Plyo Touchdown Switch

Perform a Lateral Lunge (#072) to the left, keeping your chest high as you simultaneously reach your right hand to your left toes. Push through your left foot to jump back up to the starting stance, then repeat on the opposite side. Continue quickly alternating sides.

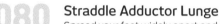

080 Straddle Adductor Lunge

Spread your feet widely apart and bend your knees. Clasp your hands in front of you and distribute your weight evenly between your feet. Bend forward at a 45-degree angle to the floor so that your hips are behind your heels. Alternate leaning from side to side.

081 Suspended Adductor Lunge

Incorporate this advanced version of an adductor lunge into your interval training only after you've mastered the Straddle Adductor Lunge (#080).

Adduction and Abduction

Your muscles and joints function in a variety of ways as you work out or just move through your daily life, and exercise names often refer to these movements. The term **abduction** refers to movement away from the body: the contraction of an abductor muscle moves a limb away from the midline of the body or from another part. **Adduction** is toward the body: the contraction of an adductor muscle moves a limb toward the midline of the body or toward another part.

- Use a TRX suspension system or loop a suspension band over a sturdy object. Stand with the anchoring point of the band at your side and place the near foot inside the looped band.

- Clasp your hands in front of you and, keeping your chest up, bend your standing leg and push your butt back as you sink down into a lunge so that the suspended leg slides out to the side as you sit back and down.

- Driving through your standing heel, return to standing, pulling the suspended leg back in toward your standing leg.

- Perform the desired reps, then repeat on the opposite side.

082

Forward Bend

Moving through daily life requires quite a bit of bending, whether you are reaching down to pick up your child or retrieving your dropped car keys. The Forward Bend and its variations prepare you to do these everyday movements with ease and efficiency, and they also get you in shape for high-intensity activities like gymnastics and martial arts. Bending exercises can strengthen muscles and joints while helping you to become more flexible by stretching and opening tight areas of your body. The Forward Bend particularly targets the hamstrings muscles and the spine.

piriformis*

gluteus maximus

gluteus medius*

erector spinae*

biceps femoris

iliopsoas*

tractus iliotibialis

gastrocnemius

soleus

Annotation Key
Bold text indicates target muscles
Black text indicates other working muscles
* indicates deep muscles

Correct form
Make the stretch long and smooth, and reach down only as far as you can comfortably extend. As you lower your torso, keep your back flat, and tuck your abdominals in toward your spine. Lengthen your spine as much as possible.

Avoid
Avoid bouncing as you reach your fingers toward your toes.

· Stand tall with your arms at your sides.

· Raise your arms toward the ceiling.

· Exhale and bend forward from your hips, sweeping your arms to the sides with your palms facing the floor.

083 Deep Forward Bend

Perform a Forward Bend (#082), and then fold your torso and abdominals onto the front of your legs, aiming your forehead toward your shins. Grasp the backs of your ankles, and contract your thigh muscles to try to straighten your knees as much as possible. Hold for the desired time, and then release.

084 Standing Split

Stand tall, then shift your weight onto your left foot. Bend forward with your back flat, simultaneously raising your right leg behind you. Square your shoulders and reach your fingertips toward the floor. Inhale, hold your right ankle with your right hand, and lift your heel toward the ceiling. Maintain balance with your right palm on the floor. Hold for the desired time, and then release. Switch sides and repeat.

085 ITB Floor Touch

Stand upright with your arms straight along your sides. Cross one foot in front of the other. Bending at your waist, gradually reach toward the floor with your hands. Hold for the desired time, and then release, slowly rolling up, and repeat twice. Switch sides and repeat.

086 ITB Forward Bend

Stand upright with your arms straight along your sides. Cross one foot in front of the other. Bending at your waist, grasp your legs at the shins. Hold for the desired time, and then release, slowly rolling up, and repeat twice. Switch sides and repeat.

Why Worry about Your Iliotibial Band?

The iliotibial tract or band, commonly known as the ITB or IT band, is a thick band of fibrous tissue that runs down the outside of the thigh, beginning at the iliac crest and extending to the outer side of the shinbone, just below the knee joint. The ITB also attaches to the gluteal muscles and the tensor fascia latae, the muscle on the outside of your hip that moves your leg outward. The ITB functions in coordination with several of the thigh muscles to extend, abduct, and laterally rotate the hip. It also contributes to lateral knee stabilization. In order to work out at high intensities—running and jumping, in particular—it is essential to keep the ITB in shape. Iliotibial band syndrome, usually shortened to IT band syndrome or simply ITBS, is common in runners, and it occurs when the ITB thickens and rubs the knee bone, producing inflammation. Certain structural factors may make you more susceptible, such as a difference in length between one leg and the other.

087 Wide-Legged Forward Bend

Stand tall, and then take a large step—about three to four feet (90 to 120 cm)—to the side. Your feet should be parallel to each other. Exhale and bend forward from your hips, keeping your back flat. With your elbows straight, place your fingertips on the floor. With another exhalation, place your hands on the floor in between your feet and lower your torso into a full forward bend, bending your elbows and placing your forehead on the floor. Hold for the desired time, and then straighten your elbows and raise your torso while keeping your back flat to return to the starting position.

088 Wide-Legged Half Forward Bend

Stand tall, and then take a large step—about three to four feet (90 to 120 cm)—to the side. Your feet should be parallel to each other. Exhale, bending forward until your torso is nearly parallel to the floor. Place your hands on the floor, making sure that your lower back is straight. Hold for the desired time and then release.

089 Alternating Toe Touches

Perform the Wide-Legged Half Forward Bend (#088), and then, keeping your back flat, touch your fingertips to your left foot. Return to standing position, and repeat on the other side. Continue alternating right and left toe touches, keeping a rapid, steady pace.

090 Seated Forward Bend

Sit on the floor as straight as possible with your back flattened and your legs extended in front of you. Lean forward, lowering your abdominals toward your thighs and extending your arms forward until you can grasp the soles of your feet with both hands.

091 Single-Leg Seated Forward Bend

Sit on the floor as straight as possible with your back flattened and your legs extended in front of you in parallel position, and then bend your right leg until it is turned out with the bottom of your right foot resting at your left inner thigh just above the kneecap. Rest your hands on your knee and bend from your waist to lean forward over your left leg. Grasp the inside of your left foot with your right hand. Use your left hand to guide your torso to the left. Return to the starting position, then repeat on the other side.

092

Side Bend

The Side Bend does a lot with a little: this simple move strengthens and stretches the spinal stabilizer muscles, including the erector spinae, latissimus dorsi, and obliques. A functional flexibility exercise, the Side Bend helps improve the performance of daily movements, like reaching into a high cabinet, or sport movements, like shooting a basketball. It will also improve your balance and general range of motion. Use it between moves during high-intensity intervals.

deltoideus posterior

latissimus dorsi

erector spinae*

obliquus externus

obliquus internus*

trapezius

teres minor

teres major

Correct form
Elongate your arms and shoulders as much as possible.

Avoid
Avoid dropping to the side too quickly—be sure to move with control

Annotation Key
Bold text indicates target muscles
Black text indicates other working muscles
* indicates deep muscles

· Stand with your feet together, keeping your neck, shoulders, and torso straight.

· Raise both arms above your head and clasp your hands together, palms facing upward.

· Leaning from your hips, drop your torso to the left.

· Return to the starting position, then lean your torso to the right. Keeping a smooth flow, continue alternating sides.

093 Side Bend Squat

Spread your feet widely apart and bend your knees into a squat. Let your arms hang straight down at your sides. Leaning from your hips and moving with control, slowly drop your torso to the right, at the same time extending your left arm straight up toward the ceiling. Return to the starting position, then lean your torso to the left while raising your right arm. Keeping a smooth flow, continue alternating sides.

094 Dumbbell Side Bend

Stand with your feet hip-width apart and your arms at your sides, a dumbbell in each hand. Leaning from your hips, drop your torso to the right, lowering the weight toward your right knee. Pause and then slowly return to the starting position, and then lean your torso to the left, lowering the weight toward your left knee. Keeping a smooth flow, continue alternating sides.

095 Dumbbell Side Crunch

Stand with your feet hip-width apart, a dumbbell in each hand. Raise your right arm straight up toward the ceiling. Lift your right knee while bending to the right to bring your right elbow and knee together, doing a side crunch. Straighten your spine as you bring your right foot to the floor, lowering your arm to return to the starting position, and then lift your left knee while bending to the left to bring your left elbow and knee together. Keeping a smooth flow, continue alternating sides.

096 Windmill

With your right arm extended along your side and your feet shoulder-width apart, stand with your left hand raised overhead. Push your left hip out to the left and slightly bend your knees while lowering your torso to the right as far as possible. Pause, then return to the starting position. Complete the desired repetitions, then repeat on the other side.

097 Kettlebell Windmill

With your right arm extended along your side and your feet shoulder-width apart, stand with a kettlebell in your left hand, then raise the weight overhead. Perform as you would a Windmill (#096).

098

Lateral Step-Over

The Lateral Step-Over is great exercise to help you improve lateral quickness and increase your agility. Perform it as a drill to really focus on your coordination, starting at half speed and, as the footwork becomes familiar, working up to moving as quickly as you can while maintaining good form. You can also vary the height and width of your obstacle—try setting up small cones or a low step to start out, eventually stepping over higher benches or steps.

- Stand next to a step or flat bench.

- Raise the knee of the leg closest to the bench and then lower your foot down to the floor on the opposite side of the bench.

- Lift the opposite leg to meet the other, bringing your feet together.

- Reverse the motion until you are standing with both feet together in the starting position. Repeat in a continuous motion for the desired time or reps.

Annotation Key
Bold text indicates target muscles
Black text indicates other working muscles
* indicates deep muscles

Correct form
Keep facing forward.

Avoid
When stepping over the bench, be sure to raise your leg, and then rotate your thigh outward—avoid just turning your torso to step over the bench.

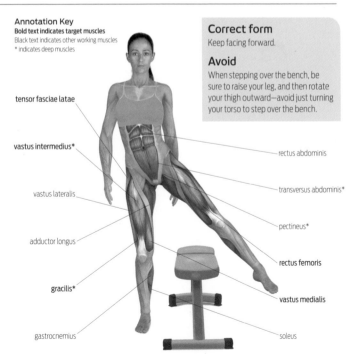

tensor fasciae latae

vastus intermedius*

vastus lateralis

adductor longus

gracilis*

gastrocnemius

rectus abdominis

transversus abdominis*

pectineus*

rectus femoris

vastus medialis

soleus

erector spinae*

gluteus maximus

obturator externus

adductor magnus

biceps femoris

semitendinosus

semimembranosus

099 Resisted Side Steps

Stand with your feet shoulder-width apart with a resistance loop or a resistance band tied around your ankles. Tuck your pelvis slightly forward, lift your chest, and press your shoulders downward and back. Keeping your head up and shoulders back, place your hands on your hips and step as far as you can sideways while keeping your knees slightly bent and your posture tall. Bring the opposite foot inward to meet the other foot, moving with control. Continue to step to the side for one to three sets of the desired repetitions, then repeat in the other direction.

100 Resisted Crossover Steps

Stand with your feet shoulder-width apart with a resistance loop or a resistance band tied around your ankles. Tuck your pelvis slightly forward, lift your chest, and press your shoulders downward and back. Step out with your left foot until you feel moderate tension in the band, and then cross your left foot over your right. Next, step your right foot in front of your left, and then step your left foot out, for a total of at least three steps with both feet to the left. Return to the starting position, then begin crossing right over left in the opposite direction. Repeat all moves for the desired sets and reps.

101

Step-Up

Annotation Key
Bold text indicates target muscles
Black text indicates other working muscles
* indicates deep muscles

gluteus maximus

biceps femoris

semitendinosus

semimembranosus

As part of a strength and conditioning program, the Step-Up effectively tones and sculpts your lower-body muscles, especially your quads, glutes, hip flexors, and hamstrings. It is also a great balance move for improving stability in your pelvis and legs, and adds a strong dose of cardio to a workout. Start with a step or box high enough that you must bend your knee to at least a 90-degree angle. Build up to higher boxes or benches as your strength and stamina improve.

Correct form
Push through the working heel, keeping that foot planted.

Avoid
Avoid hyperextending your knee past your toes or moving faster than you can while still maintaining control.

rectus abdominis

rectus femoris

vastus intermedius

vastus lateralis

gastrocnemius

vastus medialis

soleus

· Stand in front of a step or bench.

· Step onto the bench with your right leg, making sure your foot is flat on the bench.

· Lean forward slightly and push upward through the heel of your right foot, stepping up so that your left foot rests on the bench.

· Step down with your right leg, and repeat the same sequence with your left leg. Continue stepping up and down, alternating sides.

102 Alternating Step-Up with Knee Lift

Perform as you would the Step-Up (#101), but at the top of the movement when both feet are on the step, raise one knee as high as you can. Lower your knee, step down, and repeat on the other side.

103 Step-Up with Knee Lift and Overhead Extension

Perform as you would an Alternating Step-Up with Knee Lift (#102), but as you raise your knee, simultaneously extend the opposite arm straight toward the ceiling. Lower your knee and arm, step down, and repeat on the other side.

104 Dumbbell Step-Up

Holding a dumbbell in each hand with your arms at your sides, perform the Step-Up (#101). Continue stepping up and down, alternating sides for the desired reps.

105 Lateral Step and Curl

Stand with your feet hip-width apart and your arms at your sides, a dumbbell in each hand. Position a step beside your right foot. Step to the right, placing your right foot on the step. Simultaneously bend your elbows, curling the dumbbells into your chest. Lowering the dumbbells, bring your left leg onto the step. Curl the dumbbells into your chest as you step your right leg off the step. Release the dumbbells as you step down with your left leg to return to the starting position with the step to your right.

106 Curling Step and Raise

Stand with your feet hip-width apart and your arms at your sides, a dumbbell in each hand. Position a step beside your left foot. Place your left foot on the step. Shift your weight onto your left foot. Bend your elbows, curling the dumbbells toward your chest. At the same time, raise your right knee as your foot comes off the floor. Lowering the dumbbells, cross your right leg over your left leg, which should bend slightly as you lower your right leg to the floor, to the left of the platform. Simultaneously bend your left leg slightly. Step your left leg onto the floor so that you are in the starting position on the other side of the step. Repeat on the other side, and continue to alternate sides for the desired reps.

107 Medicine Ball Crossover Step-Up

Stand with your feet hip-width apart holding a Medicine ball in front of your chest. Position a high step and a lower step beside your left foot. Cross your right leg over your left, resting it on the step. Shift your weight onto your right foot to step up. Rest your left foot on the lower step. Again, cross your right leg over your left to step down onto the floor. Step your right leg onto the floor so that you are standing to the left of the step. Repeat in the other direction.

108 Crossover Bench Step-Up

Stand to the right of a bench. Cross your right leg in front of your left and step on to the bench. Push through the stabilized right heel on the bench to raise yourself up. Bring your left leg up on to the bench, then perform the motion in reverse to step down. Repeat for the desired repetitions, and then repeat on the opposite leg.

109 Side Step-Up Shuffle

Stand with your left foot on a low box or step and your right foot on the floor, about two feet (60 cm) to the right of the box. Bend your knees slightly, keep your chest up, and bend your arms to 90 degrees, keeping your elbows close to your body. Push off your left foot and jump to your left, landing with your right foot on the box and your left foot on the floor, knees bent. Push off your right foot to jump back to the starting position.

110 Side Step-Up with Lateral Leg Raise

Stand to the right of a bench or step. Step on to the bench with your right leg and push up. As you bring your left leg up, power it out to the left and raise your arms to shoulder height. Keep your focus and feet forward. Step down to the same side to complete one rep.

111 Balance Ball Triple Squat Lateral Step-Up

With the platform side down, stand to the side of a balance ball trainer with your right foot on top. Squat down, and then step onto the dome with your left foot, lowering into another squat. Next, step to the other side of the balance ball and squat, repeating the side-to-side sequence for the desired repetitions.

112

Step-Down

High-intensity workouts often call for moves that can be hard on the knees, such as jumping and running. Including exercises in your routine that strengthen the muscles that support this joint is wise. The Step-Down is particularly effective at working the vastus medialis. This muscle, one of the quadriceps, runs along the inside portion of your front thigh, closest to your kneecap. When your vastus medialis muscle is weak, it is unable to support the knee cap in proper alignment.

Correct form
Activate the vastus medialis, pushing through the ball of the foot on your working leg to keep your leg elevated throughout the contraction.

Avoid
Avoid allowing your extended knee to twist inward; instead, keep it in line with your middle toe.

adductor longus

vastus medialis

rectus abdominis

obliquus externus

transversus abdominis*

deltoideus anterior

deltoideus medialis

sartorius

gluteus medius*

tensor fasciae latae

gluteus maximus

vastus intermedius*

biceps femoris

rectus femoris

semitendinosus

vastus lateralis

semimembranosus

gastrocnemius

- Stand facing forward on a step with feet together and hands on hips.

- Bend your right leg. Simultaneously step your left leg downward, flexing the foot to rest on your heel.

- Without rotating your torso or knee, press upward through your right leg to return to the starting position. Switch legs and repeat, continuing to alternate legs for the desired repetitions.

113 Lateral Step-Down

Like the Step-Down, the Lateral Step-Down is a highly functional exercise that strengthens your muscles to prepare them for high-intensity workouts, as well as daily life. This version of a step-down move strengthens your quadriceps, along with your glutes, hip abductors, and hip adductors, and promotes the smooth coordination of your hip and leg muscles.

- Stand up straight on a step or block.

- Plant your left foot close to the edge, and allow your right foot to hang off the side.

- Flex the toes of your right foot.

- Lift your arms out in front of you for balance, keeping them parallel to the floor.

- Lower your torso as you bend at your hips and knees, dropping your right leg toward the floor.

- Without rotating your torso or knee, press upward through your left leg to return to the starting position.

- Perform the desired reps, then repeat on the other side.

114 Medicine Ball Lateral Step-Down

Grasp a Medicine ball in both hands and perform as you would the Lateral Step-Down (#113), but as you drop your right leg toward the floor, simultaneously extend the Medicine ball forward so at the bottom of the movement, the ball and your arms are fully extended from your torso and balance is achieved. Return to the starting position by extending your hip and knee and elevating your torso, while at the same time drawing the weight back toward your chest. Perform the desired reps, then repeat on the other side.

115

Toe-Up

You rely on the gastrocnemius muscles on the backs of your calves for everyday movement (especially walking) and for high-intensity activities, such as jumping and running. The shape and insertion points of these diamond-shaped muscles are largely a result of genetics, so changing the look of them through exercise can be hard, if not impossible. Yet, exercises like the Toe-Up can help you target these stubborn muscles, along with the other major calf muscle, the soleus, and keep them strong and ready for action. It can also keep your Achilles tendon supple and injury-free.

Correct form
Engage each head of your calf muscles by gently and slowly rolling from your big toe to your small toe and back again, shifting your body weight over your toes as you go.

Avoid
Bouncing to achieve a greater stretch.

Annotation Key
Bold text indicates target muscles
Black text indicates other working muscles
* indicates deep muscles

gastrocnemius

soleus

Achilles tendon

- Stand with your legs and feet parallel and shoulder-width apart in front of a step. Bend your knees very slightly and tuck your pelvis slightly forward, then lift your chest and press your shoulders downward and back.

- Position the ball of your right foot on the step.

- With your knees straight, bring your hips forward.

- Release, switch feet, and repeat on the other side.

116 Heel Drop

Stand on a step with your legs and feet parallel and shoulder-width apart. Bend your knees very slightly and tuck your pelvis slightly forward, then lift your chest and press your shoulders downward and back. Position your left foot slightly in front of your right, and place the ball of your right foot on the edge of the step. Drop your right heel down while controlling the amount of weight on the right leg to increase or decrease the intensity of the stretch in the right calf. Release, switch feet, and repeat on the other side.

117 Heel Raise

Stand with your arms at your sides (you can hold a hand weight or dumbbell in each hand with palms facing inward). Keeping the rest of your body steady, slowly raise your heels off the floor to balance on the balls of your feet. Hold for 10 seconds, lower your heels, and then continue for the desired repetitions.

118 Heel Raise with Overhead Press

The Heel Raise exercise, also known as the Calf Raise, targets the same muscles as the Toe-Up, including the gastrocnemius, soleus, and tibialis posterior of the calf. In this version, the Heel Raise with Overhead Press, you simultaneously perform an overhead pressing motion to add some upper-body emphasis to this lower-body classic.

· Stand with your feet hip-width apart and your arms at your sides, a dumbbell or hand weight in each hand.

· Raise your arms, bending your elbows and lifting your arms until the dumbbells are at ear height.

· Bring the weights overhead as you lift your heels off the floor to stand on your tiptoes. Balance for a few seconds, if desired.

· Lower your heels to the floor and bring your arms back to the starting position. Continue for the desired repetitions or time.

119

Running

Running has earned its place as a top high-intensity cardio workout that will get your heart rate up. These days there are plenty of fitness trackers with heart-rate monitors that give you the numbers you need. To determine your optimal range, first calculate your target zone by subtracting your age from 220 and multiplying by 70 percent. For example, if you are 30 years old, you would subtract 30 from 220 to get 190. You would then multiply 190 by .7 to get a target heart rate of 133 beats per minute.

Annotation Key
Bold text indicates target muscles
Black text indicates other working muscles
* indicates deep muscles

erector spinae*

serratus anterior

obliquus externus

gluteus maximus

rectus abdominis

obliquus internus*

vastus intermedius*

tibialis anterior

rectus femoris

gastrocnemius

soleus

vastus lateralis

- Stand tall and begin by warming up with a light jog, hopping from foot to foot and lifting your feet only an inch or two off the ground. To warm up your upper body, give yourself a few bear hugs.

- Begin your run with a relaxed and easy stride. Increase your pace slowly until you're running at your desired level, then lift your knees higher, alternating periods of high intensity with periods of recovery.

Correct form
Be sure to move your arms as you run—the more you move every bit of your body, the more calories you'll burn and the more effective the cardio workout.

Avoid
Avoid running in worn-out or other inappropriate footwear. If you plan to run often, get yourself fitted for a supportive pair of running shoes.

120   Skipping

Go ahead and indulge your inner child, and skip on down the road. Skipping may seem like a frivolous pursuit—and it's certainly fun—but it gives you a great cardio workout. Runners can use this activity as a dynamic warm-up session, too.

· Stand with your feet hip-width apart. With your upper arms pressed to your sides, bend your elbows to 90 degrees. Drive your right knee and left arm up while exploding upward off your left leg.

· Land on your left leg, and then immediately drive your left knee and right arm up while pushing off from your right foot.

· With each skip, propel yourself upward as high as possible and aim your knee toward your chest. Continue skipping until you have covered the desired distance.

121   Backpedaling

Stand with your feet hip-width apart. With your upper arms pressed to your sides, bend your elbows to 90 degrees. Run backward with short, quick steps, pumping your arms up and down and landing on the balls of your feet. Keep your chest up, and continue backpedaling until you have covered the desired distance.

122   Butt Kicks

Begin in a standing position, and then begin jogging in place. Kick your heels up as high as you can, aiming toward your glutes. Continue jogging and lifting your heels high, while increasing your speed until you have covered the desired distance or have run for the desired time.

123   Farmer's Walk

Stand with your feet shoulder-width apart, holding a pair of kettlebells or dumbbells in each hand with your arms by your sides. Walk rapidly for a predetermined distance or time (for example, the length of the gym or 20 seconds) while holding the weights. Lower the weights, rest, and repeat for the desired sets.

124   Monster Walk

Begin in a standing position, and then walk in place, kicking each leg out straight in front of you. As you elevate your leg, attempt to touch your foot with the opposite hand. Continue alternating sides until you have covered the desired distance or walked for the desired time.

125

High Knees

The high knees exercise combines the action of jogging in place with exaggerated knee lifts. It is a versatile move that can serve as a dynamic cardio warm-up, especially for runners—but it can help improve running form for any athlete—and it also helps build speed, power, and flexibility.

Correct form
Lift your knees as high as you can while also keeping your back and torso erect.

Avoid
Avoid pushing solely off your toes—push off from your entire foot and build up in speed as you go.

Annotation Key
Bold text indicates target muscles
Black text indicates other working muscles
* indicates deep muscles

serratus anterior

rectus abdominis

obliquus internus*

vastus intermedius*

obliquus externus

rectus femoris

vastus lateralis

semitendinosus

tibialis anterior

biceps femoris

gastrocnemius

vastus medialis

soleus

- Stand tall with your hands either on your hips or down by your sides.

- Raise up one knee as high as you are able, aiming it toward your chest, and then return to the starting position.

- Alternate legs while increasing your speed as you jog in place.

126 High Knees March

Stand tall with your feet slightly apart, your weight on the balls of your feet. Raise up one knee as high as you are able, keeping your toes up. Drive your leg back toward the floor, taking a step forward. Repeat the movement with your right leg. Continue to march until you have covered the desired distance.

127 High Knees March with Arm Raise

Perform as you would the High Knees March (#126), but as you raise your knee, extend the opposite arm overhead. Alternate sides as you march.

128 Swiss Ball Marching

Stand tall holding a Swiss ball overhead. Drive your right knee upward while lowering the ball to touch it to your knee. Drive your right leg back to the floor, taking a step forward as you raise the ball back overhead. Repeat with the left leg, and continue to march until you have covered the desired distance.

129 Steam Engine

Stand with your feet hip-width apart and interlock your fingers behind your head. Drive your right knee upward while twisting your torso to touch your left elbow to your right knee. Pause at the top of the movement, and then return your right foot to the floor. Repeat with your left leg, and continue to alternate knees until your muscles fatigue.

130 Twisting Knee Raise

Stand with your feet hip-width apart and raise both arms, bending your elbows up and facing your palms forward. Perform as you would the Steam Engine (#129), alternating knees until your muscles fatigue.

131 Knee Raise with Lateral Extension

Stand with your feet hip-width apart and your arms at your sides, a dumbbell in each hand. Shifting your weight onto your left leg, raise your right knee while lifting your arms until the weights are slightly below shoulder height. Find your balance, then, keeping your arms and upper body stationary, extend your right leg out to the side. Hold and then lower your arms, and return your right leg to the starting position. Repeat on the other side. Continue alternating sides for the desired repetitions.

132

Obstacle Course Warm-Up

Obstacle course challenges are a fun way to get your heart going while training for speed, power, agility, and coordination. You can purchase obstacle course kits that supply you with cones and discs, or you can use everyday objects like paper plates and buckets. The Obstacle Course Warm-Up starts you out with this boot camp-style training, moving you through a course of small disc training cones as you step, hop, and jog, and perform Jumping Jacks.

semitendinosus

biceps femoris

semimembranosus

rectus abdominis

vastus intermedius*

rectus femoris

vastus medialis

multifidus spinae*

gluteus medius*

gluteus minimus*

tensor fasciae latae

vastus lateralis

gastrocnemius

- Set up seven small objects on the floor to form a triangle and a square.

- Taking small, quick steps, step around all of the objects in the triangle.

- Stand in front of the square and jump forward to land in the middle of the square. Complete a Jumping Jack (#165).

- Jump forward to land outside the square. Jog back to the beginning of the course, and repeat.

Correct form
Keep a steady, measured pace as you move through the course, remaining upright throughout.

Avoid
Avoid stopping at any point, and don't take large steps; be sure to take small steps, focusing on coordination.

133 Obstacle Course Challenge

The Obstacle Course Challenge ups the intensity, adding high cones and aerobic steps to the small disc cones. You also add resistance, holding a Medicine ball as you move through the course for added strength training.

· Set up a series of cones, shorter objects, and a step on the floor as shown.

· Holding a Medicine ball in front of your chest, jump between the objects as you make your way diagonally from one corner to the other.

· Jump over one cone and then the other. Still holding the ball, challenge yourself to jump over the step.

Correct form
Keep the Medicine ball in place, centered in front of your chest. Engage your abdominal muscles and maintain a steady pace.

Avoid
Avoid twisting your neck, hunching your shoulders, moving in a jerky manner, or letting go of the ball.

134

Straight Kick

Kicking exercises can be part of a great aerobic workout and form the foundation of many high-intensity sports, like kickboxing and other forms of martial arts. Combining kicks with punches provides a full-body, calorie-burning workout and is a fantastic way to release stress. Try using kickboxing pads or punching bags to burn even more calories and to fully engage your core. To get started, try the Straight Kick (also known as the Front Kick), which will help you to learn the action and hone your balance, and then move on to more complex moves, like Roundhouse and other martial arts moves.

Correct form
Perform this kick with your upper body straight and balanced, beginning in a staggered stance. If you assume the correct starting position, you will appear to be leaning forward, and you should feel a slight stretch in your hamstrings.

Avoid
Kicking higher than you can while still maintaining good form.

- Stand with your hands on your hips in a staggered stance, with your left foot forward.

- Kick upward with your right foot, shifting your weight to your left foot as your right foot leaves the floor.

- End back in the staggered stance, and continue kicking for the desired repetitions.

- Switch sides, and continue kicking with the left foot.

iliopsoas*

pectineus*

tensor fasciae latae

sartorius

gracilis*

vastus medialis

serratus anterior

obliquus internus*

obliquus externus

gluteus maximus

biceps femoris

peroneus

tibialis anterior

adductor longus

semimembranosus

semitendinosus

adductor magnus

rectus femoris

vastus intermedius*

vastus lateralis

soleus

Annotation Key
Bold text indicates target muscles
Black text indicates other working muscles
* indicates deep muscles

135   Kick with Toe Touch

Stand with your right hand on your hip, and extend your left arm straight up toward the ceiling. Kick upward, shifting your weight to your left foot as your right foot leaves the floor. At the same time, reach your left arm to touch the toes of your right foot. Bring your right foot to the floor as your raise your right arm, and then repeat, kicking with your left leg and reaching with your right arm. Continue alternating legs, keeping a steady, smooth pace.

136   Kick with Arm Reach

Perform as you would a Straight Kick (#134), but as you raise your leg, extend the opposite arm straight out, engaging all your arm muscles. Switch sides, and continue kicking with the opposite foot. Continue alternating legs and arms.

137   Switch Kick Punch

Assume a boxing stance with your fists up, your left foot forward, your right foot back and to the right, and your knees slightly bent. Bracing your core, kick your right foot in front of you, leg straight, while punching your left fist toward your foot. Quickly return to the starting position, place your right foot in front of your left, and repeat on the other side. Continue alternating sides.

138   Martial Arts Kick

Assume a boxing stance with your fists up, your left foot forward, your right foot back and to the right, and your knees slightly bent. Raise your right knee toward your chest. Rotate your hips and left foot, and kick your right leg to the side, pushing through the heel while punching with your right arm. Quickly bring your right leg down, placing it staggered in front of your left. Bring your right arm back in. Repeat with your left leg and arm to complete one rep.

139   Roundhouse Kick

Assume a boxing stance with your fists up, your left foot forward, your right foot back and to the right, and your knees slightly bent. Pivoting slightly on your left foot, swing your right leg up, and snap your foot at the top, aiming for a waist-, shoulder-, or head-height target before bringing it down. Repeat with your left leg to complete one rep.

140

Side Kick

Like a Straight Kick, the Side Kick (also known as a Lateral Kick) works to strengthen your lower body while giving you a cardio workout and preparing you for more complex compound kick exercises. The lateral movement of your legs in this version adds emphasis to your oblique muscles.

trapezius

tensor fasciae latae

sartorius

vastus intermedius*

obliquus externus

iliopsoas

vastus lateralis

rectus femoris

tibialis anterior

infraspinatus*

subscapularis*

teres major

gluteus minimus*

piriformis*

supraspinatus*

teres minor

rhomboideus*

gluteus medius*

gluteus maximus

Annotation Key
Bold text indicates target muscles
Black text indicates other working muscles
* indicates deep muscles

Correct form
Kick straight out to the side, making sure your foot is in line with your shoulders

Avoid
Avoid jutting out your foot in front of you nor shifting it back behind you.

· Stand with feet hip-width apart and your arms at your sides.

· Kick your right leg out to the side, keeping it in line with your torso and shifting your weight to your left foot as your right foot leaves the floor. At the same time, extend both arms out to the side until they are at shoulder height, parallel to the floor.

· Return to the starting position, and repeat on the other side, then continue alternating legs.

141 Swiss Ball Side Kicks
Stand with feet hip-width apart holding a Swiss ball straight overhead. Kick your right leg out to the side, keeping it in line with your torso and shifting your weight to your left foot as your right foot leaves the floor. At the same time, bend your torso to the right, bringing the ball toward your right foot. Return to the starting position, and repeat on the other side, then continue alternating legs.

142 Round Kick
Assume a boxing stance with your fists up and your left foot forward and your right foot back and to the right. Take a small step with your left foot, pointing your left foot out, and then use your hips to swing your right leg around like a baseball bat, aiming to hit your target at thigh level. Repeat with your left leg and arm to complete one rep.

143 Side Kick Reach
Stand with feet hip-width apart. Place your left hand on your hip and extend your right arm straight up toward the ceiling. Kick your right leg out to the side, keeping it in line with your torso and shifting your weight to your left foot as your right foot leaves the floor. At the same time, reach your right arm toward your right foot. Bring your right foot to the floor as you raise your left arm, and then repeat, kicking with your left leg and reaching with your left hand. Continue alternating legs.

144

Lateral Bounding

Lateral Bounding targets several areas, including the quadriceps, hamstrings, glutes, and calves. Its principal aim is to help you practice lateral movement at speed. Try completing a set of jumps to one side, and then switching. Alternatively, add an extra level of difficulty by performing the routine while holding a Medicine ball.

Annotation Key
Bold text indicates target muscles
Black text indicates other working muscles
* indicates deep muscles

obliquus externus

rectus abdominis

transversus abdominis*

obliquus internus*

vastus intermedius*

tensor fasciae latae

vastus medialis

rectus femoris

adductor magnus

sartorius

vastus lateralis

adductor longus

soleus

gracilis*

gastrocnemius

tibialis anterior

peroneus

gluteus minimus*

gluteus medius*

gluteus maximus

semitendinosus

biceps femoris

semimembranosus

· Start in a quarter-squat position, then bound off your right foot as far and high as possible to your left. Be sure to land on your left foot.

· Next, bound as far and as high as possible back to your right off your left foot. Continue bounding from side to side.

Correct form
Be sure to keep a tight core throughout the movement. To prepare for this move, practice your lateral form by working on mastering the Lateral Lunge exercise (#072).

Avoid
Don't allow your knees to protrude far too far in front of your feet when you decelerate, land, or squat.

145 Lateral Bunny Hops

Stand tall with your feet together. Jump to the side, keeping your legs as close together as possible. Continue making small jumps side to side for the desired time or reps.

146 Lateral Shuffle

Stand with your legs open, feet placed more than hip-width apart, and bend your knees to assume a half-squat stance. Place your hands on your hips or rest them on your thighs. Stay in the squat position while bringing your left foot to your right, and then your right foot to your left. Hold the squat position while shuffling for the desired reps in each direction.

147 Side-to-Side Obstacle Springing

Set an agility cone, wire training hurdle, overturned bucket, or other object on the floor. Stand with one foot on either side of it. Spring upward with your knee high and straight. Continue springing upward, back and forth, for the desired time or reps.

148 Side-to-Side Hop

Lay a straight-line obstacle, such as a tape measure, yardstick, or a stretched-out resistance band, on the floor. Stand to the right of the line and bend your right knee to stand on your left leg. Hop sideways back and forth over the line for the desired time or reps, and then switch legs.

149 Slalom Jumps

Stand with your feet together and bend down to reach your right hand to the floor. In one motion, quickly swing both hands in front of you, elbows bent, and jump to the left, landing softly. Immediately bend your knees to reach your left hand onto the floor, and repeat the movement to the right to return to the starting position. Continue alternating sides.

150 Cone Jumps

Stand to the right of a cone. Jump off both feet to your left to clear the cone, landing on your left foot only. Put your right foot down, and leap off both feet to clear the cone again. Be sure to land on your right foot this time. Only the foot that is farthest away from the cone should make contact with the floor.

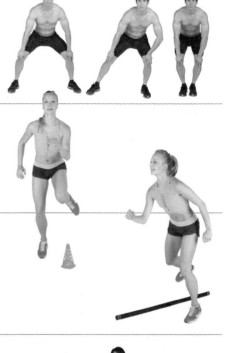

151

Jumping

biceps femoris

semitendinosus

semimembranosus

Before beginning a high-intensity workout, perform this simple move to warm up the soleus and gastrocnemius muscles of your calves, as well as to get your heart rate going. You can add jumps to just about any exercise, from squats and lunges to push-ups and squat thrusts to add a cardio burst to any workout routine.

gluteus maximus

tensor fasciae latae

gastrocnemius

vastus intermedius*

rectus femoris

tibialis anterior

vastus medialis

vastus lateralis

peroneus

soleus

Annotation Key
Bold text indicates target muscles
Black text indicates other working muscles
* indicates deep muscles

Correct form
Maintain an erect posture throughout the movement.

Avoid
Avoid landing on your toes or heels—land on the balls of your feet.

· Stand straight with your feet close together, but not touching.

· Jump up slightly, and land without touching your heels to the floor. Continue for the desired time or reps.

152 Distance Leap

Stand straight with your feet close together, but not touching. Jump from your left foot and land on your right. Then jump from your right foot and land on your left. Continue rapidly for the desired time or distance.

153 Jump to Balance Ball

Stand in front of a balance ball placed dome-side up. Drop down into a quarter-squat and then push through your heels, swing your arms, and spring up on to the dome. Land softly on your heels, and spring backward off the dome.

154 Cheer Jump

Stand with your feet together and your hands on your hips. Bend your knees into a half-squat and then jump upward as high as you can, bending both legs at the knee to bring your feet back and up toward your glutes. As you jump, bring your arms over your head into a V position. Continue without pause for the desired amount of time or repetitions.

155 Depth Jumps

Face two plyo boxes or platforms placed about three feet (1 meter) apart from each other, and then stand on top of the one closest to you. Jump off the box, making sure to land on the balls of your feet between the two boxes. As soon as your feet hit the floor, spring up on to the other box. As soon as you land on the second box, turn around, and repeat in the other direction.

156 Tuck Jumps

Stand with your knees slightly bent and your elbows bent to 90 degrees. Bend your knees into a half-squat and then jump straight upward by bending slightly forward and tucking your knees upward to touch your elbows. Land on the balls of your feet, and continue jumping up and down without pause for the desired amount of time or repetitions.

157 Stadium Jumps

Stand at the base of a staircase that has steps at least as deep as the length of your feet. Drop down into a quarter-squat, then push through your heels, swing your arms, and spring up to the first step. Find your balance, and then spring to the next, finding a steady, well-balanced rhythm.

Plyometric Boxes and Aerobic Steps

A sure way to add intensity to your workout is to work with boxes and steps—just think of the long-standing popularity of step aerobics classes to burn calories and elevate heart rate. In functional training and boot camp gyms, many lower-body exercises call for you to jump on and off a box or step, which can help you to increase your speed, power, and explosiveness. When choosing a box, look for sturdy construction and a variety of sizes—adjustable models and sets are available that generally range in height from 12 to 30 inches (30 to 76 cm) high. Aerobic steps and platforms can vary in height, too. Look for stackable versions that you can adjust, depending on your workout or fitness goals.

158 Step Jumps

Stand in front of an aerobic step or low box. Bend your knees into a quarter-squat, then push through your heels, swing your arms forward, and spring up on to the step. Land softly on your heels, and then quickly spring backward off the step. Continue without pause for the desired amount of time or repetitions.

159 Box Jumps

Stand in front of a plyo box or other platform. Bend your knees into a quarter-squat, then push through your heels, swing your arms, and spring up on to the box. Land softly on your heels, and then step down. Continue for the desired time or reps.

160 Straddle Box Jumps

Stand with your feet on either side of an aerobic step or low box. Bend your knees into a quarter-squat, then push through your heels, swing your arms forward, and spring upward to land with both feet on the first step. Find your balance, and then jump as high as possible while spreading your legs as wide as you can as you bring your arms forward. Land on the balls of your feet, returning to the starting position with your feet on either side of the step. Continue without pause for the desired amount of time or repetitions.

161

Skipping Rope

Skipping, or jumping, rope, may be a schoolyard favorite, but like many a childhood activity, it is a high-energy exercise that really burns calories. Athletes, such as boxers, and military personnel are known for skipping rope as a training move, and it is an effective exercise to perform as a rest between other exercise sets to recover your heart rate.

deltoideus medialis

deltoideus anterior

biceps brachii

vastus intermedius*

rectus femoris

vastus lateralis

soleus

vastus medialis

gastrocnemius

Annotation Key
Bold text indicates target muscles
Black text indicates other working muscles
* indicates deep muscles

- Stand with the jump rope in your hands, letting the rope hang behind your feet.

- Swing the rope around your body and jump over it. Keep your arms as straight as you can during the movement, and land with both feet together on the floor.

Correct form

Begin with the right rope. To judge the proper length, stand on the middle of the rope—the handles should extend to your armpits. To begin the exercise, hold the rope with your hands at about hip height with your elbows slightly bent. Keep your upper arms close to your sides as you swing the rope with your chest out and your shoulders back and down.

Avoid

Avoid jumping too high; keep your jumps small, and make sure to land on the balls of your feet.

Star Jump

As many a special forces candidate or high-school cheerleader can attest, the Star Jump is harder than it looks—you must be able to jump high enough to simultaneously extend your legs and arms outward. To develop leg strength and cardiovascular endurance, as well as improve bone density, you can challenge yourself to perform as many as you can in quick succession, being sure to concentrate on maintaining perfect form.

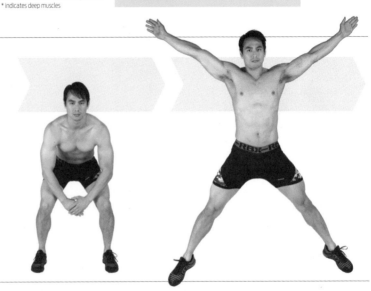

biceps brachii

deltoideus anterior

triceps brachii

rectus abdominis

obliquus externus

obliquus internus

rectus femoris

vastus intermedius

vastus lateralis

vastus medialis

erector spinae

gluteus maximus

obturator externus

adductor magnus

biceps femoris

semitendinosus

semimembranosus

Annotation Key
Bold text indicates target muscles
Black text indicates other working muscles
* indicates deep muscles

Correct form
Flare out your legs as far as possible, while making sure not to twist in the jump; landing in an awkward position could cause a torque injury. Also be sure to jump on a soft surface, such as an exercise mat or padded carpeting, to reduce the landing impact.

Avoid
Avoid landing on your toes or heels—land on the balls of your feet.

· Stand with your feet together and then squat down, keeping your knees in line with your toes.

· In one explosive movement, jump as high as possible while spreading your arms and legs as wide as you can. Your body will make a star shape at the fully extended point of the jump.

· Bend your knees slightly as you land in a standing position. Sink back to a squat, and repeat. Each jump equals one repetition.

163 Straddle Leap

Stand with your feet together and your arms at your sides. Bend your knees, squatting down completely to the floor with your heels slightly raised. Place your hands on the floor for balance, look upward, and then push off the floor to jump straight up. At the peak of the jump, pop your legs out to the sides, straighten your arms, and reach for your toes. Land softly on the balls of your feet, and continue without pause for the desired amount of time or repetitions.

164 Stag Leap

Stand with your feet together. Bend your knees, and then jump upward as high as you can, bending both legs at the knee and wrapping your back leg around your body, with your knee parallel to the floor. As you leap, lift your arms over your head. Land softly on the balls of your feet, and continue without pause for the desired amount of time or repetitions.

165 Jumping Jack

Stand with your feet together, arms extended with your hands at your sides. Bend your knees slightly and push through the balls of your feet as you straighten your knees to jump upward while spreading your legs as wide as you can. At the same time, raise both arms out and up in a smooth arc. As you return to the floor, bring your feet together and your hands back to your sides. Continue without pause for the desired amount of time or repetitions.

166 Jumping Jack Clap

Perform as you would a Jumping Jack (#165), but at the top of the movement, sharply clap your hands together. Continue without pause for the desired amount of time or repetitions.

167 Scissor-Stance Jacks

Stand with your left foot in front of your right with your knees slightly bent and fists raised in front of you. Bracing your core, kick your right foot in front of you, leg straight, while punching your left fist toward your foot. Quickly return to the starting position, place your right foot in front of your left, and repeat on the other side. Continue alternating without pause for the desired amount of time or repetitions.

168

Skater

The high-energy Skater targets your inner and outer thighs, including your hip adductor and abductor muscles and iliotibial bands, which all work to keep your knees and hips stable. Try it if you are a runner: it counterbalances the effects of repetitive flexion and extension, alleviating the resulting strength imbalance between the inner- and outer-thigh muscles and the quadriceps and hamstrings.

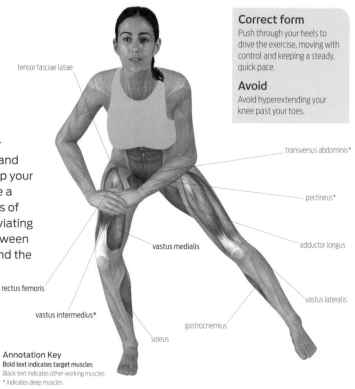

tensor fasciae latae

transversus abdominis*

pectineus*

adductor longus

vastus medialis

vastus lateralis

rectus femoris

vastus intermedius*

gastrocnemius

soleus

Correct form
Push through your heels to drive the exercise, moving with control and keeping a steady, quick pace.

Avoid
Avoid hyperextending your knee past your toes.

erector spinae*

gluteus minimus*

gluteus maximus

adductor magnus

biceps femoris

semitendinosus

semimembranosus

Annotation Key
Bold text indicates target muscles
Black text indicates other working muscles
* indicates deep muscles

- Stand with your legs spaced wider than shoulder-width apart and your toes pointing forward.

- Slide to your side into a side lunge as you bend forward slightly with your hands placed on your thigh, and then move in the opposite direction.

- Slide back and forth for the desired time or repetitions.

169 Dumbbell Skater

Grasp a dumbbell in each hand and perform the Skater (#168) while curling the dumbbells upward as you move from side to side.

170 Straight-Leg Skater

Stand straight and place your left leg slightly behind your right. Keeping your legs and back straight, jump to your left as far as possible while swinging your arms toward the left. Land in a standing position with your right leg slightly behind your left. Continue jumping side to side, crossing one leg behind the other. Switching back and forth equals one repetition.

171 Speed Skater

Stand in a half-squat position and place your left leg slightly behind your right. Jump to your left as far as possible while swinging your arms toward the left. Land in a half-squat position with your right leg slightly behind your left. Immediately jump back toward the right as far as possible, as if you were skating in long strides. Continue to alternate sides for the desired amount of time or repetitions.

172 Step Skater

Stand with your right foot on an aerobic step with your left foot planted at least a foot from the step. Extend your arms out at shoulder height. Bend forward at the hip, reaching down to touch your right foot with your left hand. Rise back up, placing both feet on the step, and then drop your right foot to the floor. Bring your right hand to your left foot. Bring both feet back to the step, and then repeat all steps, continuing to alternate sides for the desired amount of time or repetitions.

173

Swimming

A functional move that is also a Pilates staple, the Swimming exercise can strengthen your core muscles while improving your coordination and endurance. As your strength improves, keep increasing the speed and tempo of your strokes.

Correct form
Stretch your limbs out as far as possible. Tightly squeeze your glutes, and draw your navel into your spine throughout the exercise.

Avoid
Tensing your neck or lifting your shoulders toward your ears.

- Lie prone on the floor with your legs hip-width apart. Stretch your arms beside your ears on the floor. Engage your pelvic floor, and draw your navel into your spine.

- Extend through your upper back as you lift your left arm and right leg simultaneously. Lift your head and shoulders off the floor.

- Lower your arm and leg to the starting position, maintaining a stretch in your limbs throughout.

- Extend your right arm and left leg off the floor, lengthening and lifting your head and shoulders. Continue to alternate arms and legs for the desired repetitions.

Annotation Key
Bold text indicates target muscles
Black text indicates other working muscles
* indicates deep muscles

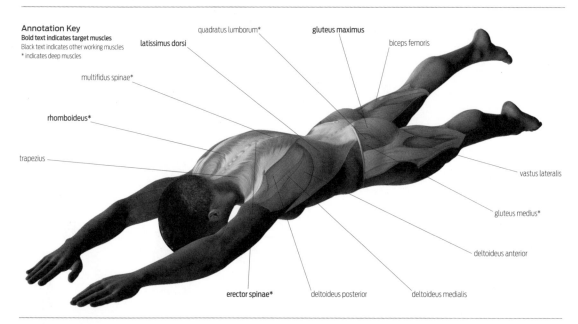

quadratus lumborum*

gluteus maximus

latissimus dorsi

biceps femoris

multifidus spinae*

rhomboideus*

trapezius

vastus lateralis

gluteus medius*

deltoideus anterior

erector spinae*

deltoideus posterior

deltoideus medialis

174 Arm Hauler

Lie facedown with your arms spread wide, keeping them level with your shoulders. Lift your head, keeping your chin up while arching your lower back. Bring your arms off the floor and reach behind you as far as your can. Without letting your hands touch the floor, bring your arms forward to touch your fingertips together. Draw your arms back to the starting position and continue for the desired repetitions.

175 Facedown Snow Angel

Lie facedown on the floor with your legs hip-width apart. Lift your arms and legs at the same time, and move them as if you were making snow angels.

176 Superman

Lie prone on the floor with your legs hip-width apart. Lift both arms and legs simultaneously, continuing to draw your navel into your spine.

177 Heel Beats

Work your hamstrings, glutes, inner thighs, lower back, and lower abs all while lying prone. This Pilates staple will also boost your coordination and endurance.

- Lie facedown with your arms lifted off the floor by your hips with your palms up. Draw your shoulders down, away from your ears. Turn your legs out from the top of your hips and pull your thighs together.

- Lengthen your legs and lift them off the mat, tightening your thigh muscle. Press your heels together and then separate them in a rapid but controlled motion.

178 Weighted Ball Heel Beats

Lie facedown with your forearms on the floor. Rest your hips on top of a weighted ball. Extend your legs behind you. Press your heels together, and then separate them in a rapid but controlled motion.

179 Supine Flutter Kicks

Lie on your back with your arms stretched along the sides of your body. Keeping your heels a few inches off the floor, kick up and down, alternating legs.

180

Bear Crawl

The Bear Crawl is a favorite of military special forces around the world, helping to train recruits for real-world movements. Crawling exercises can be tough, but they are great for increasing agility, cardiovascular health, and upper-body strength. They are anaerobic exercises, meaning that they trigger lactic acid formation, which promotes strength, speed, and power.

pectoralis minor*

deltoideus anterior

biceps brachii

pectoralis major

triceps brachii

Correct form
Move as steadily and as smoothly as possible.

Avoid
Avoid placing all of your weight on your arms and shoulders, which can stress your rotator cuffs. Don't let your knees touch the floor.

· Place both hands and feet on the floor.

· Walk your left arm and right leg forward, and then your right arm and left leg.

· Keep moving forward and backward in this position, keeping your weight evenly distributed between your arms and legs.

181 Alligator Crawl

Start in the drop position, with your hands directly below your shoulders. Lower into a half push-up with your back straight. Keeping your body low to the floor, bring your right knee to your right elbow while walking your left hand forward. Reverse this movement by walking your right hand forward and bringing your left knee to your left elbow. Continue moving forward, reversing your hand and knee positions for the desired time.

182 Crab Crawl

Begin with both hands and feet on the floor. Lift your body slightly so that your butt is just above the floor. Walk your right foot forward, then walk your left foot forward. Continue moving forward, taking several steps with each leg. Next, walk each leg back. Alternate moving backward and forward for the desired time.

183 Inchworm

Stand straight, arms at your sides. Bend forward from the waist and place your hands on the floor in front of you, at a distance slightly wider than your feet. Keep your knees as straight as possible. Shift your weight to your hands, and slowly "walk" them forward while keeping your knees straight, your hips up, and your spine straight. Return by walking back toward the starting position and pushing your hips upward, folding your torso at the hips. This exercise is also called the Hand Walk-Out.

Mountain Climber

Correct form
Keep your back straight, and flare your hands out to ease shoulder stress.

Avoid
Don't make small movements with your legs; attempt to bring each knee to your chest for each count.

A favorite of military special forces, the Mountain Climber exercise is a high-intensity move that gets your heart rate going while it challenges the muscles of your legs and core. This compound exercise helps to develop muscular endurance in your arms, as well as hone your balance, agility, proprioception, and coordination. Keep a steady pace by moving to a 1–2 count.

gluteus maximus
vastus intermedius*
rectus femoris
vastus lateralis
gastrocnemius
deltoideus anterior
biceps brachii
triceps brachii
deltoideus medialis

- With your hands shoulder-width apart, place your palms on the floor, keeping your feet together and back straight. Push your body up until your arms are straight. This starting position is the high plank, or drop position.

- Bring your right knee in toward your chest, and rest the ball of your foot on the floor for count 1.

- Jump, and bring your left knee to your chest for count 2. Continue alternating your feet as fast as you can safely go for the desired time or repetitions, keeping pace by counting 1–2, 1–2.

185 Cross-Body Mountain Climber

Assume the drop position with your body straight and core tight. Pick up one foot and bring your knee toward the opposite shoulder. Return to the starting position, then quickly alternate legs.

186 Balance Ball Mountain Climber

Place a balance ball dome-side down and get into a high plank position on it with your shoulders directly over your wrists. Keeping your hips in place and your core tight, bring one knee toward your chest, then quickly alternate legs.

187 Spider Mountain Climber

Assume a low plank position with your shoulders over your elbows. Bend one leg and bring your knee as close to your same-side shoulder as you can. Take it back down and repeat on the other side.

188 Sliding Mountain Climber

Place a sliding disc, paper plate, or small towel under each foot. Assume the high plank position with your hands just wider than shoulder-width apart. Bring one knee toward your chest, pulling the sliding disc, then quickly alternate legs.

189 Swiss Ball Mountain Climber

Place your hands on a Swiss ball, and then extend your legs behind you in the high plank position. Raise one foot, and slowly bring your knee toward your chest, then lower it. Repeat with the other leg, and continue alternating legs as you try to keep the ball in place.

190 Fire Hydrant Mountain Climber

Assume a low plank position with your shoulders over your elbows and then drive your knee forward, out, and up, aiming to get your thigh parallel to the floor and your knee as far forward as possible.

191 Suspended Mountain Climber

Loop two suspension bands over a sturdy object. Place your feet in the loops, then assume a high plank position, facing away from the anchor point with your hands under your shoulders and one leg pulled up to your chest. Alternate pulling your knees toward your chest.

192

Mountain Climber with Hands on Desk or Bench

Assume the drop position with your hands on top of a bench and your feet planted firmly on the floor. Keep your arms fully extended and directly beneath your shoulders. Brace your core, and drive one knee to the mid-line of your body. Reverse the motion, and step your foot back to the starting position.

193

Resistance Band Mountain Climber

Loop or tie a resistance band loosely around your ankles. Assume the drop position, and then perform as you would a Mountain Climber (#184).

194

Slalom Skier

Assume the drop position. Jump both feet together to the left so that both feet land outside your left arm. Tuck your knees toward your chest as you jump. Jump your feet back to the leaning rest position, and then jump both feet back across your body to the right, landing with both feet outside your right arm and both knees bent toward your chest. Immediately jump back to the left, and continue alternating sides. Both left and right equal one repetition.

195

Plank Bunny Hop

Lay a straight-line obstacle, such as a pole, tape measure, yardstick, or stretched-out resistance band, on the floor. Assume the drop position with one hand on each side of the line and both feet to the left of it. Jump both feet forward so that your calves are parallel to the floor, forming a right angle with your thighs. In one explosive movement, jump both feet to the right, lifting your body as high as you can. Land on the balls of both feet, and then immediately jump to the other side. Continue jumping back and forth over the line without pause for the desired amount of time or repetitions.

196

Diagonal Reach

As simple as it may look, the Diagonal Reach trains multiple muscles at once—especially your abdominals and obliques. This exercise, along with the Medicine Ball Over-the-Shoulder Throw is a multipurpose move that helps you to develop balance, coordination, and power while stabilizing and strengthening your core.

Annotation Key
Bold text indicates target muscles
Black text indicates other working muscles
* indicates deep muscles

coracobrachialis*

pectoralis major

pectoralis minor*

obliquus internus*

iliopsoas*

deltoideus anterior

deltoideus medialis

deltoideus posterior

rectus abdominis

erector spinae*

obliquus externus

rectus femoris

Correct form
Keep your abdominal muscles engaged throughout the movement, with your hips facing forward and your shoulders pressed down.

Avoid
Avoid twisting your hips, hunching your shoulders, or tensing your neck as you lift or lower your arms.

- Stand with your feet hip-width apart and your arms at your sides.

- Raise both arms upward and to the right to form a diagonal line. Follow your hands with your gaze. Return to the starting position.

- Repeat to the left side.

197 Over-the-Shoulder Throw

Working with a weighted ball during the Over-the-Shoulder Throw adds resistance and force to the Diagonal Reach movement, and, like that exercise, it has multiple benefits, helping you to improve your balance and coordination while stabilizing and strengthening your core. You can perform it with a partner, taking turns to throw the ball to each other, or you can perform it facing a wall.

Correct form
Keep your abdominal muscles engaged throughout the movement, your hips squared and your shoulders pressed down.

Avoid
Avoid hunching your shoulders or tensing your neck as you lift or lower your arms.

· Stand with your feet hip-width apart holding a weighted ball in your hands at waist height. Extend your arms forward and rotate your core, moving your extended arms slightly upward and to the side so that the weighted ball follows your body's twist.

· Twist your torso in the other direction as you raise your arms in an arc. At the top of the arc, with your torso twisted, release the ball to your partner.

· Lower your arms and return your torso to the center, and then retrieve the ball. Perform the desired repetitions, and then switch sides.

198

Figure 8

The Figure 8 exercise is both a core stabilizer and a core strengthener. It is great for anyone who wants to build rotational power, such as baseball pitcher or golfer. You can experiment with form and speed when performing this move—the bigger you make the 8s, the more of a challenge it will be. Try upping your speed too, while still keeping good form.

Correct form
Move through the exercise as quickly as you can while still maintaining control using your core.

Avoid
Don't let the momentum of the ball drive your movements.

Annotation Key
Bold text indicates target muscles
Black text indicates other working muscles
* indicates deep muscles

deltoideus anterior
deltoideus posterior
rectus abdominis
obliquus externus
obliquus internus*

· Stand with your feet hip-width apart and your arms at your sides.

· Raise both arms upward and to the right to form a diagonal line. Follow your hands with your gaze. Return to the starting position.

· Repeat to the left side.

erector spinae
biceps femoris
semitendinosus
semimembranosus

199 Cable Woodchop

Stand with your feet slightly wider than hip-distance apart, with a cable weight machine to your right. Grasp the handle of the cable in both hands. With your legs slightly bent, smoothly rotate your core and raise your arms diagonally to the upper right toward the cable machine. In a controlled chopping motion, bring your arms diagonally back to the starting position and then down to the other side, rotating your core away from the machine. Complete the desired number of repetitions, then repeat in the opposite direction.

200 Waist-Height Woodchop

Perform a Cable Woodchop (#199), bringing the cable to just shoulder height. This offers you a chance to focus on your form without straining your arm muscles.

201 Twisting Lift with Body Bar

Stand with your feet planted hip-distance apart and your arms stretched out holding a body bar at shoulder height. With a smooth movement, bend your elbows to bring the bar toward your chest, keeping your elbows near shoulder height. Using your hips as a hinge, turn to the right side, keeping your arms stationary and slightly bending your left knee. Gradually twist back to face forward. Straighten your arms to return to the starting position. Complete the desired number of repetitions, then repeat in the opposite direction.

202 Big Circles with Medicine Ball

Stand with your feet hip-width apart or slightly wider, holding a Medicine ball above your head, with your arms straight. Swing your arms downward and to the side, keeping your arms straight throughout the movement. Continue swinging the ball to the opposite side and up in a continual 360-degree circular motion. Complete the desired number of circles, then repeat in the opposite direction.

Why Use a Medicine Ball?

A Medicine ball is a useful piece of fitness equipment—you can hold it or lift it as you would a dumbbell to add resistance to an exercise, and you can toss it, slam it, or pass it to add explosive power to a move. It allows you to work in all three planes of motion —frontal (forward and back), sagittal (side to side), and transverse (up and down), and it is great for working on strength, stability, balance, and coordination. Medicine balls come in a wide variety of sizes and weights, from small 2-pound (900 g) versions to enormous 150 pounders (68 kg). You can also choose from hard versions to softer bouncing balls, as well as ones with handles or ropes and water-filled varieties. For the most stable grip, be sure to hold a Medicine ball with your hands open and fingers spread wide.

203 Kettlebell Figure 8

The Kettlebell Figure-8 is a strength builder, primarily of the trunk and hips. Strength, coordination, timing, and accuracy are required to perform this exercise correctly.

- Assume a wide stance and hold a kettlebell in your right hand between your legs, close to your right thigh.

- Bend forward slightly, keeping your back flat and pushing out your buttocks.

- Bring the kettlebell toward your left leg and receive it in your left hand, which should come from behind the left leg.

- Repeat the movement with the left hand, switching the kettlebell from in front of the left leg to the right hand behind the right leg. This forms a figure 8 around your static legs.

- Continue passing the kettlebell between your legs to form the 8s for the desired time or repetitions, and then switch directions. Instead of switching hands, swing the kettlebell back out with the same hand and back in front of the same leg it just circled around. Perform the desired number of passes.

Correct form
Look for controlled repetitions as you keep your back flat, and move your hips side to side during the movement

Avoid
Avoid excessive speed, bouncy repetitions, and shallow or incomplete passes.

204 Hand-Clap Figure 8

Assume a wide stance, and then bend forward slightly, keeping your back flat and pushing out your buttocks. Moving your hips to the left, bring your hands behind your left leg, and clap sharply. Then move your hands and your hips to the right and clap behind your right leg. Continue moving back and forth, forming figure 8s for the desired time or repetitions, and then switch directions.

205

Medicine Ball Throw

The Medicine Ball Throw takes a real-world movement—throwing—and adds the explosive power of a Medicine ball to provide rotational drive that can help you build stamina and core stability.

deltoideus anterior

deltoideus medialis

rectus abdominis

deltoideus posterior

obliquus externus

obliquus internus*

gluteus medius*

rectus femoris

gluteus minimus*

vastus medialis

gluteus maximus

gastrocnemius

vastus lateralis

Annotation Key
Bold text indicates target muscles
Black text indicates other working muscles
* indicates deep muscles

- Hold a weighted Medicine ball in front of your chest, taking a few steps forward to get ready.

- Prepare to throw the ball by positioning your left foot behind you with the heel off the floor. Keeping your torso stable, raise the ball until it is positioned above your right shoulder.

- Bend the knee of your back foot to lift it off the floor as you throw the ball forward.

- Retrieve the ball, and then repeat on the opposite side. Continue for the desired time and repetitions.

biceps femoris

semitendinosus

semimembranosus

Correct form
Engage your abdominal muscles as you throw.

Avoid
Avoid excessively twisting your torso to either side—make sure to keep your torso facing forward.

206 Weighted Ball Throw and Catch

The Weighted Ball Throw and Catch is another functional move that builds stamina and core stability. Perform this exercise with a buddy, each of you executing alternating motions as you toss the ball back and forth between you.

- Stand facing your partner, holding a weighted ball behind your head.

- Raise the ball over your head and forward in a sweeping throwing motion, and then release the ball to your partner.

- Receive the returned ball and repeat, with each partner alternating throwing and catching.

207 Weighted Ball Slam

Stand upright, holding a weighted ball behind your head with elbows bent. Swing the ball over your head and slam it straight down with force, squatting as you do so. Catch the ball in the squat position. Stand up, and repeat.

208 Wall Ball

Holding a weighted ball below your chin, face a wall at arm's length distance. Stand with your legs and feet parallel and shoulder-width apart and your knees bent very slightly. Tuck your pelvis slightly forward, lift your chest, and press your shoulders down and back. Lower into a squat, and then forcefully stand up, throwing the weighted ball upward at an overhead target on the wall. Continue squatting and throwing for the desired time.

High-Intensity Functional Training

Wall Balls, Box Jumps, Kettlebells Swings . . . high-intensity exercises like these have taken gyms by storm as functional training and boot camp-style programs have risen in popularity. The most well-known of these may be CrossFit®, a branded fitness regimen created by Greg Glassman, which, according to the company, is a strength and conditioning program consisting of "constantly varied functional movements executed at high intensity across broad time and modal domains." CrossFit gyms and others with similar programs use a range of fitness techniques and equipment, including weights (like barbells, dumbbells, kettlebells, and Medicine balls), gymnastics rings, pull-up bars, jump ropes, plyo boxes, and resistance bands. The regimen changes regularly, with workouts of the day (WODs) a feature. Wall Balls are often included because this grueling exercise works so many muscles—including your abs, glutes, quads, hamstrings, calves, lower back, chest, deltoids, biceps and triceps—and increases your overall power and explosive strength.

209

Power Punch

You don't have to step into the ring to reap the benefits of boxing, which is a great way to incinerate calories, build strength, and boost stamina. To get the most out of this high-intensity, high-energy kind of workout, you need to get to know the basic fighting stance and punches: the jab, cross, uppercut, and hook. Exercises like the Power Punch lay the groundwork so that you can go on to practice combo moves. You can perform punching exercises alone (in other words, shadowboxing) or you can work with punching bags or a sparring partner.

trapezius

deltoideus medialis

erector spinae*

latissimus dorsi

obliquus externus

obliquus internus*

deltoideus anterior

deltoideus posterior

rhomboideus*

serratus anterior

rectus abdominis

Annotation Key
Bold text indicates target muscles
Black text indicates other working muscles
* indicates deep muscles

· Stand with your feet shoulder-width apart and one leg placed slightly in front of the other, with most of your weight on your back leg. Keep your elbows in and raise your fists up. This is the basic fighting stance.

· Transferring your weight to your front leg, punch straight in front of you with the fist closest to your body as you turn your torso in to lend power to the punch.

· Punch for the desired time or repetitions, and then reverse sides, switching both arms and legs.

Correct form
Keep your fists up and rotate your torso to drive the movement.

Avoid
Avoid sloppy form or excessive speed—maintain a steady, even, but modest pace.

210 Dumbbell Cross Jab

Stand with your feet a bit wider than hip-width apart and your knees very slightly bent. Hold a dumbbell in each hand at chest height with your elbows bent and palms facing each other. Extend your left arm across your body until the weight is in line with your right shoulder. As you return to the starting position, repeat with the right arm. That's one rep. Punch for the desired time or reps, continuing to alternate arms.

211 Uppercut

Stand with your feet shoulder-width apart and one leg placed slightly in front of the other, with most of your weight on your back leg. Keeping your elbows in, raise your fists and punch upward toward the sky as you rotate your torso and transfer most of your weight to your front foot. Punch for the desired time or reps, and then reverse sides, switching both arms and legs.

212 Jump Cross

Stand with your feet hip-width apart, your knees bent and your fists raised to shoulder height. Jump upward, raising your arms overhead. As you land, pivot to the left, and punch your right fist straight out in front of you. Quickly return to the starting position, and repeat on the other side, pivoting to the right and punching with your left fist. Continue alternating sides for the desired time or reps.

213

Battle Rope Side-to-Side Swings

The rising popularity of rope training comes as no surprise. Working with these simple tools provides you with powerful strength training and high-energy cardio and helps you to build speed and agility. Battle rope exercises particularly target your core and upper body, with a strong contribution from your lower-body muscles. Moves like the Battle Rope Side-to-Side Swings also call for your obliques to kick in. Whatever moves you choose, battle ropes offer an efficient way to build lean muscle (without heavy weights), while torching calories and upping your heart rate.

rectus abdominis
deltoideus anterior
deltoideus medialis
biceps brachii
obliquus externus
obliquus internus*
vastus lateralis
rectus femoris
vastus medialis

trapezius
deltoideus posterior
triceps brachii
latissimus dorsi
erector spinae*

Annotation Key
Bold text indicates target muscles
Black text indicates other working muscles
* indicates deep muscles

· Stand with your knees slightly bent and take a battle rope in each hand. Bring your hands together, keeping the ropes around waist height.

· Brace your core. In one motion, forcefully swing the ropes to the left. Reverse the motion, bringing the ropes to the right.

· Continue swinging the ropes from side to side while maintaining a strong, tight, and braced stance.

Correct form
Engage your abdominals throughout the exercise.

Avoid
Don't pull the rope tight: you want enough slack so it can move smoothly.

gluteus maximus
biceps femoris
semitendinosus
semimembranosus
gastrocnemius

214 Battle Rope Alternating Waves

Stand with your knees slightly bent, holding the ends of the rope at arm's length in front of your hips with your hands shoulder-width apart. Tuck your elbows into your sides and brace your core, and then begin alternately raising and lowering each arm explosively. Keep alternating arms for the desired time.

215 Full-Squat Alternating Wave

Holding a battle rope in each hand, bend your knees and drive your hips back while bracing your core to assume a full squat position. Bring the left rope up as you move the right rope down, and then immediately bring the right rope up and the left rope down. Keep repeating this alternating motion while remaining in the squat position for the desired time.

216 Jump Squat and Slam

Holding a battle rope in each hand, bend your knees and then drive your hips back while bracing your core to assume a full squat position. Explosively jump as high as you can. When you land, immediately squat down, then jump again. Continue squatting and jumping for the desired time, then finish by slamming the rope down. Keep repeating this motion for the desired time.

217 Snakes

Stand with your knees slightly bent and take a battle rope in each hand. Bring your hands together, keeping the ropes around waist height. Brace your core and then move the rope in and out close to the floor to create two symmetrical zigzags.

218 External-Rotation Spirals

Stand with your knees slightly bent and take a battle rope in each hand, starting with your hands at your sides. Circle each arm outward (never inward) to create two symmetrical spirals.

219 Battle Claps

Stand with your knees slightly bent and take a battle rope in each hand. Bring your hands together, keeping the ropes around waist height. Brace your core and then move your arms in and out, as if you were clapping your hands together.

220 Crossover Slam

Stand with your knees slightly bent and take the ends of a battle rope in each hand. Bring your hands together and then move the ends of the ropes in an arc above your head, lifting them to your left and then slamming them down hard to your right while keeping both feet flat on the floor. Repeat in the opposite direction. Keep alternating sides for the desired time or repetitions.

221 Battle Jacks

Stand with your knees slightly bent and take the ends of a battle rope in each hand, starting with your hands at your sides. Forcefully push off the floor into a small jump and extend your legs to each side to land with your feet spread wide. At the same time, bring the ropes up above your head. Jump again, bringing your feet together and moving your arms back down toward your hips. Repeat the movement, mimicking a traditional Jumping Jack (#165).

222 Double-Arm Wave

Stand with your knees slightly bent, holding the ends of the rope at arm's length in front of your hips with your hands shoulder-width apart. Tuck your elbows into your sides, brace your core, and then pump your arms up and down together, creating waves in the ropes. Continue for the desired time or repetitions.

223 Double-Arm Slam

Stand with your knees slightly bent and take the ends of a battle rope in each hand. Lift both ends of the rope overhead, as high as you can, and then slam the rope down to the floor with as much force as you can generate. Continue lifting and slamming, going as fast as possible.

224 Double-Arm Slam Jump

Stand with your knees slightly bent and take the ends of a battle rope in each hand. Brace your core, then, in an explosive movement, bring the ropes upward to shoulder level as you perform a small jump in the air. At the top of the movement, immediately come down into a squatting position and slam the ropes downward to the floor. Repeat the movement, being sure to maintain the rope's pattern. Continue for the desired time or repetitions.

225 Grappler Throes

Stand with your knees slightly bent and take a battle rope in each hand, grasping it so that the ends are sticking out from between your thumb and index fingers. Bring the ends down next to your right hip. Keeping both feet grounded, pivot your torso to the left. During the pivot, flip the ropes over your hip, as if you were throwing a grappling opponent to the ground. Pivot back to the other side, switching back and forth for the desired time.

Battle Rope Training

Once only found at military boot camps, in martial arts gyms, and on football training fields, battle ropes have emerged into the mainstream. And with good reason—these thick, heavy, woven cables are effective tools to help build full-body strength and provide intense cardio exercise. The ropes are anchored to a wall or beam and used in pairs in what are vigorous and relatively low-impact workouts. If you want to work with them outside the gym, they are now readily available in rubber-tipped nylon, which are easiest to keep a grip on with sweaty hands.

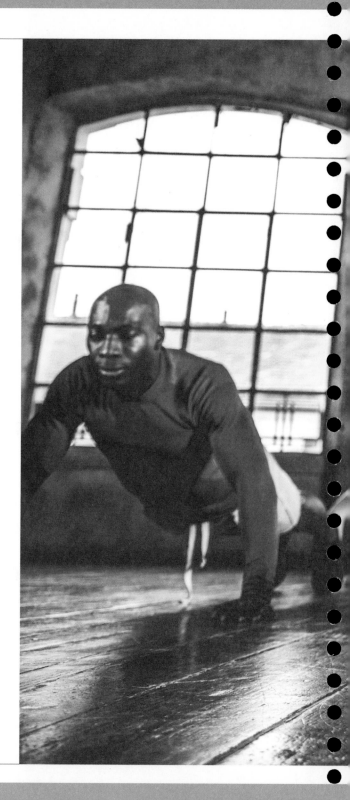

CHAPTER TWO

Power Exercises

Traditional exercises, like the push-up, pull-up, or crunch, have earned their places in both military boot camps and boot camp-style gym classes because they are so versatile—while you're working to pump up your muscles, you can also pump up your power and endurance. You can easily incorporate these classic exercises into an interval training program, performing them at high intensity and high volume to really get your heart rate up and challenge your stamina and endurance. You can also combine them with other power moves or functional exercises—the high-intensity Burpee and its many variants, for example, mixes a squat thrust with a variety of aerobic and strength moves, like jumps, push-ups, and pull-ups.

Basic Push-Up

From boot camps to school gyms, anywhere you find serious exercisers, you'll find the push-up. This classic move is used to assess fitness levels, and it is a fundamental component of military basic training. It can be a basic strength exercise, but it also serves as the foundation of many high-energy moves and can be combined with other exercises to amp up its intensity. Its "drop" starting position—legs extended and arms straight—is the launching point for numerous power exercises. Push-ups target the pectorals, triceps, and anterior deltoids, while also benefiting the midsection.

Correct form
Look for low and controlled repetitions, and keep your torso stabilized and your upper body straight. At the lowest point, your upper arms should be parallel to the ground.

Avoid
Avoid excessive speed, shallow or bouncy repetitions, or allowing your lower back to dip too far.

- With your hands shoulder-width apart, place your palms on the floor, keeping your feet together and back straight. Push your body up until your arms are straight. This is your "drop" starting position.

- Bend your arms and lower your torso until your chest touches the floor. Straighten your arms to rise back up to the starting position to complete the repetition. Perform for the desired sets and reps.

deltoideus posterior

deltoideus medialis

latissimus dorsi

obliquus externus

obliquus internus*

rectus abdominis

deltoideus anterior

pectoralis minor*

pectoralis major

biceps brachii

rectus femoris

brachioradialis

triceps brachii

Annotation Key
Bold text indicates target muscles
Black text indicates other working muscles
* indicates deep muscles

227 Knee Push-Up

Begin on your hands and knees, and then walk your hands forward, dropping your hips so that your body forms a straight line from shoulders to knees. Perform as you would a Basic Push-Up (#226). This easier version shortens the lever, reducing your lifting load by about half.

228 Wide Push-Up

Assume the drop position with your hands spaced wider than shoulder width. This hand position will take your shoulder and chest muscles through a different range of movement than a Basic Push-Up (#226), isolating the lateral part of the pectoralis major.

229 Triceps Push-Up

Assume the drop position with your hands placed close together, and perform as you would a Basic Push-Up (#226). This hand position shifts the emphasis from the pectorals to the deltoids and triceps.

230 Decline Push-Up

Begin on your hands and knees with your hands about shoulder-width apart, and then prop your feet on an elevated surface. With your back flat, bend your elbows to touch your chest to the floor, and then extend your arms back to the upright position. The decline angle applies greater pressure to the upper chest and front deltoids and isometrically contracts the core muscles.

231 Swiss Ball Decline Push-Up

Begin on your hands and knees with your hands about shoulder-width apart. Prop your toes on a Swiss ball and perform as you would a Decline Push-Up (#230).

232 Diamond Decline Push-Up

With your hands placed together so that your thumbs and index fingers touch, rest the tops of your feet on an elevated surface and perform as you would a Decline Push-Up (#230).

233 Medicine Ball Decline Push-Up

Begin on your hands and knees with your hands about shoulder-width apart. Balance your toes on a Medicine ball and perform as you would a Decline Push-Up (#230).

234 Incline Push-Up

Assume the drop position with your hands placed slightly wider than shoulder-width apart on an elevated surface. Keeping your body straight, bend your arms and lower your torso until your chest touches the surface. Pause, and then push back to the starting position. The incline angle places more emphasis on the lower chest and triceps.

235 Medicine Ball Knee Push-Up

Begin on your hands and knees with your hands on a Medicine ball. Perform as you would an Incline Push-Up (#234). Performing on a slightly unstable surface calls for increased contributions from the rotator cuff and shoulder stabilizers, which can help improve shoulder function.

236 Medicine Ball Push-Up

Assume the drop position with your hands on a Medicine ball, and perform as you would an Incline Push-Up (#234).

237 Swiss Ball Incline Push-Up

To add an element of instability, assume the drop position with your hands on a Swiss ball, and perform as you would an Incline Push-Up (#234).

238 Foam Roller Push-Up

To add an element of instability, assume the drop position with your hands on a foam roller, and perform as you would an Incline Push-Up (#234).

239 Balance Ball Push-Up

To add an element of instability, assume the drop position with your hands on the flat side of a balance ball, and perform as you would an Incline Push-Up (#234).

240 Balance Ball Diamond Push-Up

Place both hands on the rounded side of a balance ball, positioning them close together so that your thumbs and index fingers touch. Perform as you would an Incline Push-Up (#234).

241 Weighted Ball Push-Up

To add an element of instability, assume the drop position with each hand grasping a small weighted ball, and perform as you would an Incline Push-Up (#234).

242 Pilates Magic Circle Push-Up

Place the ring on the floor with the bottom pad down. Rest your sternum on the pad and your hands on the floor. Push down on the pad with your sternum until you can squeeze your upper arms against your ribcage, and then, step both feet back to come into the drop position. Perform as you would a Basic Push-Up (#226).

243 Knuckle Push-Up

Clench your fists by wrapping your thumbs around the outside of your curled index and middle fingers and assume the drop position. Perform as you would a Basic Push-Up (#226). This version is a great option for those with wrist issues, and it also allows for a slightly deeper range of motion.

Maximize Your Push-Ups

You can perform push-ups with a variety of weighted props, from standard dumbbells to specially designed push-up bars. These add-ons increase your range of motion, letting you go down slightly deeper, and they make the movement a little easier on your wrists. To perform, grasp the prop and move up and down as you would during the Basic Push-Up (#226). You can also increase resistance by adding weight, such as performing push-ups with a sandbag or plate on your back.

244 Dumbbells

247 Rotational Stands

245 Kettlebells

248 Yoga Block

246 Hand Weights

249 Sandbag

250 Weighted Santana Push-Up

The Weighted Santana Push-Up, also called a Handstand or T-Stabilization Push-Up, is a great way to combine a strength exercise and a rotational movement. This push-up variation will rev up your metabolism and increase balance and coordination.

· Assume the drop position, with your hands grasping a set of dumbbells. Bend your arms, and lower your torso until your chest touches the floor.

· Straighten your arms and, at the top of the push-up, lift your right arm straight up, rotating your torso to stack your shoulders and turning your heels to the left so that your body and arms form a T.

· Lower the right dumbbell to the floor and push off your feet, rotating your whole body in the opposite direction as you jump up. Land on your feet facing the opposite direction. This counts as one rep. Repeat all steps, this time raising your left arm.

251 Santana Push-Up

Stand with your feet hip-width apart. Squat down and put your hands on the ground in front of you. Jump your feet back into the drop position and bend your arms, lowering your torso until your chest touches the floor. Straighten your arms and, at the top of the push-up, lift your right arm straight up, rotating your torso to stack your shoulders and turning your heels to the left so that your body and arms form a T. Lower your raised hand to the floor and return to the drop position. Push off your feet, and rotate your whole body in the opposite direction as you jump up. Land on your feet facing the opposite direction. This counts as one rep. Repeat all steps, this time raising your left arm.

252 Push-Up with Lower-Body Rotation
Assume the drop position and then rotate your lower body with either your feet split and your bottom foot forward or with one foot on top of the other. Perform as you would a Basic Push-Up (#226).

253 Single-Leg Knee Push-Up
Begin on your hands and knees and then walk your hands forward, dropping your hips so that your body forms a straight line from shoulders to knees. Raise one leg, and perform as you would a Knee Push-Up (#227).

254 Single-Leg Push-Up
Assume the drop position, raise one leg, and perform as you would a Basic Push-Up (#226).

255 Single-Leg Decline Push-Up
Begin on your hands and knees with your hands spread wide, and then prop your feet on an elevated surface. Raise one leg and, with your back flat, bend your elbows to touch your chest to the floor, and then extend your arms back to the upright position.

256 Single-Leg Roller Push-Up
Begin on your hands and knees with your hands spread wide, and then prop your feet on an elevated surface. Raise one leg and, with your back flat, bend your elbows to touch your chest to the floor, and then extend your arms back to the upright position.

257 Push-Up on Swiss Ball and Blocks
With your hands shoulder-width apart and fingertips parallel to your collarbone, place your hands on blocks. Place your feet with your ankles fixed at 90-degree angles and toes down on a Swiss ball so that your body is horizontal. Bend your elbows to lower your torso until your chest is level with your hands. Return by extending your elbows and pushing into the blocks, elevating your entire body simultaneously.

258 Single-Leg Push-Up on Swiss Ball and Blocks
Keeping the toes of one foot on a Swiss ball, elevate your other leg. Perform as you would a Push-Up on Swiss Ball and Blocks (#257).

259 Box Push-Up

Place one hand on the floor and the other on a box. Bend your arms, and lower your torso until your chest is level with the box. Press forcefully back to the starting position.

260 Crossover Box Push-Up

Place your left hand on the box and your right on the floor. Perform as you would a Box Push-Up (#259), and then lift your right hand and place it beside your left hand on top of the box. Move your left hand down to the floor so your hands are shoulder-width apart. Perform another push-up to complete the repetition.

261 Single-Arm Push-Up

Assume a drop position with your legs spread wide. Bring one arm behind you to rest on the small of your back. Lower with control, turning your torso slightly away from the supporting arm so that your working arm and both feet form a triangle. When your chin is about a fist's width above the floor, push your body upward to the starting position.

262 Single-Arm, Single-Leg Push-Up

Assume the drop position and perform as you would the Basic Push-Up (#226), but at the top of the movement, raise your opposite leg and arm, pause, and then lower your arm and leg to the starting position.

263 Dynamic Box Push-Up

Assume the drop position with your hands placed closed together on a box so that your thumbs and index fingers touch. Lower your body, and then press explosively off the box, your hands landing on the floor on either side of the box. Immediately lower your body and then press up explosively so that your hands land back on the box in the starting position to complete the repetition.

264 Alternating Shuffle Push-Up

Assume the drop position and then move your right hand to the left until both hands are next to each other. Now slide your left hand farther left until your hands are shoulder-width apart again. Do a push-up, and then repeat the process, moving to the right and doing another push-up.

265 Alternating Medicine Ball Push-Up

Assume the drop position with one hand on the floor and the other hand on top of a Medicine ball. Lower your torso toward the floor, pause, and then press back up to the starting position. Roll the Medicine ball beneath the other hand before repeating the movement.

266 Push-Up with Clap

Lie flat on the floor, facedown. Place your hands slightly outside your shoulders and your fingertips parallel to your collarbone, so that your elbows are at 45-degree angles to your torso. Place both feet on tiptoes. Keeping your body rigid, forcefully and quickly push your hands into the floor so that you generate enough momentum to come off the ground. Just as your body reaches its highest point, clap your hands directly beneath your chest, and immediately return them to the floor, supporting yourself so that the rest of your body decelerates to a position just above the floor.

267 Plyo Kettlebell Push-Up

Assume the drop position with one hand planted on the floor and the other gripping a kettlebell. Lower yourself until your upper arms are parallel to the floor. Next, quickly push your arms to full extension. As you do so, switch hands on the kettlebell. Lower yourself again, switching sides each time you push yourself back up.

268 Dive Bomber

The Dive Bomber is a high-intensity plyometric push-up variation that places a lot of body weight on the shoulders and arms. The sliding position of the body mimics a bomber aircraft diving toward the ground and then swooping back up.

· Assume the drop position with your hands placed shoulder-width apart.

· Grounding your toes into the floor, walk your hands toward your feet until your butt is up in the air and your shoulders are above and slightly behind your hands.

· Lower your chest toward the floor while keeping your butt in the air.

· Arch your lower back and push your body weight out in front of your arms. Elevate your chest and straighten your arms. Reverse this movement to the starting position.

Correct form
Flex your back forward on the way down and arch it on the way up.

Avoid
Don't pause at the top or bottom of the move. To boost its cardio benefits, make the motion smooth and continuous.

269 Knee Push-Up and Roll-Out

Place a barbell on the floor so that the bar is horizontal to your torso. Grasp the bar with your elbows extended, your arms straight, and the bar beneath your chest. With your body rigid, bend your knees to the floor. Keeping your elbows at 45-degree angles to your torso, use your knees as a fulcrum and let your body drop until your chest touches the bar. Extend your elbows, and push up and away until your arms are fully extended. Pause. then push on the bar, rolling it forward with your arms remaining extended. Pause briefly, then pull back on the bar, returning it to the starting position.

270 Push-Up and Roll-Out

Perform as you would a Knee Push-Up and Roll-Out (#269), but with your legs extended and your body rigid.

271 Suspended Push-Up

Loop a suspension band over a sturdy object. Place your feet in the loop, positioning them directly under the anchor point, and assume the drop position with your feet together, your back flat, and your core tight. Bend your arms and lower your torso until your chest touches the floor. Straighten your arms to rise back up to the starting position to complete the repetition.

272 Suspended Atomic Push-Up

Loop a suspension band over a sturdy object. Place your feet in the loop and kneel facing away from the anchor point. Place your hands slightly wider than shoulder-width apart on the floor and lift up to the drop position. Bend your elbows to 90 degrees to lower your body toward the ground. Press back up, lifting your hips slightly, and crunch, bringing your knees to your chest.

273 Balance Beam Push-Up

To challenge both your strength and balance, mount a balance beam and assume the drop position with one foot stacked on the other. Take a firm grip on the beam and perform as you would a Single-Leg Push-Up (#254).

274 DFRB

This high-intensity multiphase agility exercise comes straight from special forces boot camp training grounds. "DFRB" stands for Drop, Face, Recover, and Back. "Drop" means to get into a starting push-up position. "Face" means to lower your body until your chest touches the floor. "Recover" means to jump both feet to your chest, and quickly stand up. "Back" means to flip onto your back. To perform this exercise, you move through these four positions in rapid succession. Begin by performing them in DFRB order, but as you develop strength and endurance, you can repeat the moves in any order, keeping in mind that performing all four equals one repetition.

- Stand tall with your arms at your sides.

- Drop forward into a push-up position.

- Lower your chest to the floor to assume the Face position.

- Rapidly jump both feet forward to your chest, so that you are in a full squat position.

- To assume the Back position, quickly drop your body to the floor and lie back, with your head landing where your feet were in the Face position.

- Quickly stand up. This is the Recover position.

- Jump to your feet, then repeat the DFRB sequence in any order.

275 Towel Fly

The Towel Fly is an advanced modification of a push-up that calls for you to move your arms in and out rather than up and down. Utilizing your body weight, it gives your chest muscles an efficient workout while also recruiting the muscles of your arms, back, hips, and abdomen to keep your body stabilized. Try to perform as many as 20 in a row for a high-intensity challenge. You can use a single towel, two small towels, or even paper plates under your hands—anything that will slide smoothly on the floor.

· Place a towel on the floor in front of you. Assume the drop position with your elbows fully extended and a towel under your hands.

· Maintaining a rigid drop position with your abdominals braced and your weight on your feet, move your hands together. The towel should bunch together below your sternum.

· Straighten out the towel by pressing outward with your arms, returning to the starting position.

276 Single-Arm Forward Slide

On a smooth flat surface (preferably wood), assume the drop position with legs straight and each hand placed on a small individual towel. Bend one elbow and simultaneously slide the other hand upward, keeping that elbow straight to cause your torso to descend. Return by pushing into the floor with the bent arm and pulling downward with the overhead, straightened arm until your torso returns to the starting position. Alternate arms.

277 Single-Arm Forward Knee Slide

Assume a bent-knee drop position with a towel under your knees and perform as you would the Single-Arm Forward Slide (#276).

278

Up-Down

The Up-Down exercise gets your blood pumping and the fat burning. This multiphase exercise is meant to tax your cardiovascular system by working almost all of your muscles, and it has the added benefit of increasing your agility and coordination. You can add another element of upper-body conditioning by performing the Up-Down with Push-Up variation (#279). Sport teams and military personnel rely on these exercises to develop nimbleness and speed.

deltoideus anterior

deltoideus medialis

deltoideus posterior

latissimus dorsi

triceps brachii

obliquus internus*

obliquus externus

rectus femoris

vastus lateralis

pectoralis minor*

pectoralis major

biceps brachii

vastus intermedius*

vastus medialis

rectus abdominis

Annotation Key
Bold text indicates target muscles
Black text indicates other working muscles
* indicates deep muscles

Correct form
Keep your knees at waist level while running in place.

Avoid
Avoid landing on your chest—allow your hands to contact the floor first and then lower onto your chest. Don't just flop to the floor—move with control.

• Run in place, bringing your knees waist-high with each step.

• Drop down and touch your chest to the floor.

• Immediately stand back up and resume running with high knees as quickly as possible. Perform for the desired reps and sets.

279

Up-Down with Push-Up
Perform as you would an Up-Down (#278), but when you drop down to touch your chest to the floor, raise your torso to perform a push-up. Immediately jump back up to your feet and resume running with high knees.

280

Alternating Renegade Row

Annotation Key
Bold text indicates target muscles
Black text indicates other working muscles
* indicates deep muscles

- trapezius
- deltoideus posterior
- rhomboideus*
- erector spinae*
- latissimus dorsi

Correct form
Keep your hips level and square to the floor, and fully engage your core muscles.

Avoid
Avoid jerky movements; move smoothly with control.

The Alternating Renegade Row is a hard-working exercise that combines the benefits of an explosive upper-body move with a powerful core strengthener.

- deltoideus anterior
- triceps brachii
- quadratus lumborum
- deltoideus medialis
- obliquus externus
- transversus abdominis
- pectoralis minor*
- biceps brachii
- rectus abdominis
- pectoralis major

- With a kettlebell in each hand, assume the drop position.

- While staying on your toes, pull the kettlebell in your right hand up toward your chest while straightening your left arm and pushing that kettlebell into the floor.

- Lower your right arm, then repeat with the left. Continue alternating sides for the desired repetitions.

---

281 Single-Arm Renegade Row
Perform an Alternating Renegade Row (#280), but perform all reps on one side and then repeat on the other side.

---

282 Single-Leg Renegade Row
Perform as you would the Alternating Renegade Row (#280), but raise one leg off the floor.

---

283 Single-Arm T-Row
Start in the drop position, taking a wide stance with your legs and holding a kettlebell in each hand. Pull one of the bells to chest level. Rotate your torso while raising your arm toward the ceiling. Slowly lower the kettlebells back to the floor to return to the drop position. Repeat with the other arm to complete one repetition.

Crane Handstand

Annotation Key
Bold text indicates target muscles
Black text indicates other working muscles
* indicates deep muscles

The Crane Handstand, also known as the Crane or Crow Pose, is a foundational arm-balancing yoga pose. It strengthens your upper arms, forearms, and wrists while also strengthening your abs and stretching your upper back and groin. Mastering this move improves balance and coordination—your goal is to pull your knees up near your armpits and lift your butt as high as possible while remaining balanced enough to keep your full weight off your wrists. For any handstand moves, until you have the strength and skill, working with a spotter is essential.

infraspinatus* · rhomboideus* · trapezius · teres major · deltoideus posterior · triceps brachii · biceps brachii · brachialis · extensor digitorum · brachioradialis

Correct form
To help quell a fear of falling, keep your breath even and your mind calm.

Avoid
Don't allow your head's weight to shift towards your hands.

pectoralis major · sternocleidomastoideus · serratus anterior · deltoideus anterior · coracobrachialis* · rectus abdominis · obliquus internus* · obliquus externus · transversus abdominis* · pectineus* · iliopsoas*

- Squat deeply until your buttocks are just above your heels. and then lean your torso forward and extend your arms to place your hands on the floor in front of you. Turn your hands inward slightly and widen your fingers.

- Bend your elbows, resting your knees against your upper arms. Lifting up on the balls of your feet and leaning forward with your torso, bring your thighs toward your chest and your shins to your upper arms. Round your back as you feel your weight transfer to your wrists.

- Exhale and slowly lift your feet off the floor one at a time. Keep your head position neutral and find your balance point.

285 Side Crane Handstand

Squat until your buttocks are just above your heels. Place your left hand flat on the floor outside your right thigh. Place the outside of your right thigh on your left upper arm. Lean to the right to place your right hand flat on the floor so that your hands are shoulder-width apart. Slowly lift your pelvis as you shift your weight toward your hands, using your left arm as a support for your right thigh. Continue shifting to the right, keeping your feet together as you raise them off the floor. Hold for the desired time, and then exhale as you bring your feet to the floor. Repeat on the other side.

286 Crane Handstand Push-Up

To add a further balance challenge, perform a Crane Handstand (#284) on push-ups bars.

287 Handstand

Stand straight and raise your arms over your head. Kick out with your dominant leg, and as you fall into a lunge position, tip your body forward. Hold your arms straight and move your head toward the ground. Straighten your legs and torso toward the sky, balancing your weight on your hands. To release the handstand, split your legs and drop your dominant leg to the ground. Start to stand up, and as you do, put your other leg on the ground.

288 Handstand Walk

Perform a Handstand (#287), and then walk your hands forward while maintaining balance.

289 Parkour Vault

Approach an obstacle, such as a railing, in a direct line. Reach one arm forward, place your hand flat on the top of the obstacle, and shift your weight off your feet onto your shoulder. Launch your body off the ground and kick your outer leg sideways as you vault over the obstacle. Reach your bottom foot to the floor, release your hand, and continue stepping forward. Repeat in the opposite direction, leading with your other arm.

Parkour Training

One of the most intense forms of fitness training has to be Parkour, a high-energy discipline inspired by military obstacle course training. The goal: practitioners must move through a complex obstacle-filled course as efficiently and quickly as possible using no equipment. Commonly performed as an urban acrobatic workout, Parkour moves include vaults, rolls, jumps, handstands, and swings.

290

Bench Dip

The classic Bench Dip is a medium-intensity strength move that target the triceps. Like many strength moves, it can easily be incorporated into a high-intensity workout. You can do it just about anywhere and on any elevated surface, from a flat bench at the gym, the park bench in the square, or the storage bench in your living room. A slightly more difficult version of this exercise, the Triceps Dip, calls for you to lift your entire body weight, increasing the demand on your triceps.

deltoideus anterior

obliquus externus

latissimus dorsi

deltoideus posterior

triceps brachii

deltoideus medialis

gluteus maximus

Correct form
This is an easy move to master, but it can be hard on the shoulders, so be sure to keep your movements smooth and controlled.

Avoid
Avoid allowing your feet to slide, and don't let your hips sag.

pectoralis minor*

coracobrachialis*

pectoralis major

serratus anterior

rectus abdominis

- Sit up tall near the front of a sturdy chair. Place your hands beside your hips, wrapping your fingers over the front edge of the chair.

- Extend your legs in front of you slightly, and place your feet flat on the floor. Scoot off the edge of the chair until your knees align directly above your feet and your torso will be able to clear the chair as you dip down.

- Bending your elbows directly behind you, without splaying them out to the sides, lower your torso until your elbows make a 90-degree angle.

- Press into the chair, raising your body back to the starting position.

291 Triceps Dip

Begin standing in front of a dip station or parallel bars. Place one hand on each bar and grip as you push and extend your arms to full lockout. Lower yourself until your upper arms are parallel to the ground, then push back up to the starting position.

292 Assisted Bench Dip

Perform as you would a Bench Dip (#290), placing your feet directly in front of your torso and planting them firmly on an assist bench or other platform.

293 Roller Triceps Dip

Sit on the floor with your legs outstretched, a foam roller behind you. Place both hands on the roller with your fingers facing toward your buttocks and elbows bent. Press through your legs and straighten your arms to lift your hips and shoulders. Keeping your shoulders pressed down, bend your elbows and dip your trunk up and down. The foam roller should not move.

294 Single-Leg Bench Dip

Perform as you would a Bench Dip (#290) with one leg lifted straight out, parallel to the floor, and your knees squeezed together. Perform the desired repetitions, then switch sides.

295 Floor Dip

Sit with your feet flexed in front of you and your heels touching the floor. Place your hands on the floor next to you so that your fingertips point towards your hips and your elbows point behind you. Lift your hips off the floor until your shoulders are directly over your wrists and your arms are nearly straight. Bend your elbows and dip your torso up and down without letting your buttocks touch the floor.

296 Single-Leg Floor Dip

Perform as you would a Floor Dip (#295) while keeping one leg elevated and extended straight out in front of you. Switch sides, and repeat.

297 Dip to Kick

Perform as you would a Floor Dip (#295), but at the top of the movement, kick one leg up while reaching for your toes with the opposite hand. Switch sides, and repeat.

Upward Plank

Correct form

Activate your core and gluteal muscles to hold the position. Keep your shoulders above your wrists and lengthen your spine, neck and arms.

Avoid

A void performing this exercise if you have shoulder or wrist mobility problems.

The Upward Plank is known by many names—Reverse Plank, Incline Plank, Inclined Plane, and Upward Plane. A basic back-bending yoga pose, it strengthens your core, shoulders, arm, wrist, and leg muscles. It also stretches your shoulders, chest, and ankles while helping you to hone your balance and flexibility.

· Sit with your legs extended and place the palms of your hands on the floor with fingers facing forward.

· Move your hands behind your hips, draw your knees toward your chest, and place your feet on the floor with your heels about a foot (30 cm) away from your butt.

· Press down with your hands and feet and lift your hips until your back and thighs are parallel to the floor with your shoulders directly above your wrists.

· Without lowering your hips, straighten your legs one at a time. Push your hips higher by lifting your chest and bringing your shoulder blades together, creating a slight arch in your back. Gently elongate your neck and let your head drop back.

· Hold for the desired time, and then return to the starting position.

Annotation Key
Bold text indicates target muscles
Black text indicates other working muscles
* indicates deep muscles

sternocleidomastoideus
pectoralis major
pectoralis minor*
rectus abdominis
obliquus internus*
obliquus externus
transversus abdominis*
adductor magnus
biceps femoris
gastrocnemius
scalenus*
levator scapulae*
trapezius
triceps brachii
extensor digitorum
extensor carpi radialis
deltoideus medialis
deltoideus anterior
erector spinae*
gluteus maximus
gluteus medius*

299 Upward Plank Kick

Sit with your legs parallel and stretched out in front of you. Place your hands behind you with your fingers pointed toward your hips. Press up through your arms and lift your chest, squeezing your buttocks and lifting your hips while pressing your heels into the floor. Continue lifting your pelvis until your body forms a long line from your shoulders to your feet. Without allowing your pelvis to drop, raise your right leg straight up. Slowly lower your leg to the floor, then switch to the left leg. Continue alternating legs for the desired repetitions.

300 Upward Plank Hip Lift

Place an aerobic step behind you and sit with your legs parallel and stretched out in front of you. Place your hands behind you on the step with your fingers pointed toward your hips. Lift your hips slightly so that your butt is a few inches above the floor. This is your starting position. Press up through your arms and lift your chest, squeezing your buttocks and lifting your hips while pressing your heels into the floor. Continue lifting your pelvis until your body forms a long line from your shoulders to your feet. Pause, then lower yourself back to the starting position and repeat for the desired repetitions.

301 Upward Plank March

Perform as you would the Upward Plank Kick (#299), but instead of keeping your raised leg straight, bend it to a 90-degree angle. Alternate lifting and lowering your knees as if you were marching, using a 4-count rhythm to keep a steady pace. Continue marching for the desired time or repetitions.

302

Forearm Plank

The Forearm Plank is an isometric, or contracted, exercise, designed to work your entire core. There are many versions of the plank, and they are performed everywhere from yoga and Pilates studios to hard-core gyms for a good reason: they are a reliable way to build endurance in your abs and back as well as in the core stabilizer muscles.

- Lie on your stomach with your legs extended behind you. Bend your arms so that your forearms rest flat on the floor. Keep your palms flat or make fists.

- Bend your knees, supporting your weight between your knees and your forearms. Push through with your forearms to bring your shoulders up toward the ceiling as you straighten your legs.

- With control, lower your shoulders until you feel them coming together. Hold for the desired time.

trapezius
infraspinatus*
supraspinatus*
teres minor
subscapularis*
rhomboideus*
erector spinae*

Annotation Key
Bold text indicates target muscles
Black text indicates other working muscles
* indicates deep muscles

Correct form
Fully engage your abs.

Avoid
Don't allow your butt to rise or sink.

gluteus maximus
vastus intermedius*
obliquus internus*
obliquus externus
deltoideus posterior
vastus lateralis
deltoideus anterior
gastrocnemius
serratus anterior
pectoralis minor*
tibialis anterior
rectus femoris
transversus abdominis*
rectus abdominis
pectoralis major

303

Forearm Plank Leg Extension
Assume the Forearm Plank position (#302), and then lift and lower your legs one at a time. Keep the rest of your body still, and your abs engaged throughout.

304 Forearm Plank Knee Drops

Assume the Forearm Plank position (#302) and, keeping your hips level and parallel to the floor, flex your right knee toward the floor as you inhale and extend it again as you exhale. Alternate sides for the desired repetitions.

305 Chaturanga

From the High Plank position (#314), open your chest and broaden your shoulder blades while tucking in your tailbone. With your legs turned slightly inward, lower yourself to the floor until your upper arms are parallel to your spine. Tuck your tailbone under and draw your abdominals in toward your spine to maintain the straight line from your shoulders to your heels.

306 Suspended Forearm Plank

Loop a suspension band over a sturdy object. Facing away from the anchor point, place your toes in the loop and press your forearms flat on the floor. Keeping a tight core, press your feet into the foot cradles and lift up into a plank position. Continue as long as you can maintain a perfect plank.

307 Spiderman Plank

Assume the Forearm Plank position (#302). Keeping your body in a straight line, bring your right knee to your right elbow. Hold, return to the starting position, and repeat with the left leg. Continue alternating legs for as long as you can while maintain proper form.

308 Arm-Reach Plank

Assume the Forearm Plank position (#302). Engage your abdominals and lift your right arm off the floor. Hold for the desired time and then release to return to the starting position. Switch arms and repeat.

309 Plank-Up

Assume the Forearm Plank position (#302) and then lift up with your right arm until it is fully extended. Then straighten your left arm until you are balanced on both arms in a High Plank (#314). Reverse one arm at a time, lowering from the planted hand to forearm until back in the initial Forearm Plank. Repeat for the desired repetitions, trying to maintain a steady rhythm as you move from one arm to the other.

310 Swiss Ball Forearm Plank

Position yourself on your toes with your arms bent and your forearms resting on top of a Swiss ball. Form a long, straight line from your ankles to your shoulders. Hold this position for as long as you can.

311 Swiss Ball Loop Extension

With a resistance loop or a resistance band tied around your ankles, assume the Forearm Plank position (#302) with your arms propped on a Swiss ball. Keeping your abs tight, exhale then squeeze your glutes to raise your right leg, lengthening your body as your weight transfers from your arms to your left foot. Return your right foot to the floor. Repeat for the desired reps, switch legs, and repeat on the other side.

312 Balance Ball Spiderman Plank

Assume the Forearm Plank position (#302) with your arms propped on the dome side of a balance ball. While keeping your body in a straight line, bring your right knee to your right elbow. Hold for one second, return to the starting position, and repeat with the left leg. Continue alternating legs for as long as you can while maintaining proper form.

313 Forearm Plank Roll-Down

Stand with your weight equally distributed between your feet. Bend from your waist to place your hands flat on the floor in front of your feet. Walk your hands away from your feet until your body reaches the Forearm Plank position (#302), forming a straight line from your shoulders to your heels. Keeping your arms straight, dip your shoulders three times. Walk your hands back to your feet, and return to an upright position. Perform the desired reps at a rapid pace.

314 High Plank

The High Plank is the same as a push-up's "drop" starting position—you prop your elongated body on your extended legs and straight arms. Like the drop position, it is the launching point for numerous power exercises, and in yoga, the High Plank is a base position from which you move into many other poses.

· With your hands shoulder-width apart, place your palms on the floor, keeping your feet together and back straight.

· Push your body up until your arms are straight. Hold for the desired time.

315 High Plank with Leg Extension

Assume the High Plank position (#314) with your shoulders directly over your hands and your torso straight. Lift your left leg straight toward the ceiling. Return to the High Plank and repeat with the other leg.

316 High Plank Knee Pull-In

Assume the High Plank position (#314) with your shoulders directly over your hands, your torso straight. Draw your left leg upward toward your chest. Return to the High Plank and repeat with the other leg.

317 Plank Roll-Down

Perform as you would a Forearm Plank Roll-Down (#313), walking your hands out to the High Plank position (#314) instead of the Forearm Plank.

318 High Plank Knee Pull-In with Extension

Assume the High Plank position (#314) with your shoulders directly over your hands and your torso straight. Draw your left knee into your chest, flexing the foot while rocking your body forward over your hands. You should come up on the toes of your right foot. Extend your left knee backward, rocking the body back and shifting your weight onto your heel. With your head in between your hands, straighten your right leg and lift it toward the ceiling.

319

Swiss Ball Shin Plank

This version of a plank on a Swiss ball is slightly easier than a forearm version. The Swiss Ball Shin Plank is still an effective exercise, helping to stabilize and strengthen your core, back, shoulders, and chest muscles. It also forms the foundation of many other plank moves, preparing you for higher intensity exercises.

· Kneel on your hands and knees with a Swiss ball behind you. Raise your legs to rest your shins and ankles on the ball.

· Push the ball back to lift and straighten your knees until your body forms a straight line from shoulders to feet.

· Hold this position for as long as possible, while still maintaining good form.

Correct form
To challenge yourself, prop as little of your legs on the ball as possible.

Avoid
Don't allow your middle back to sag.

quadratus lumborum*
latissimus dorsi
erector spinae*
deltoideus posterior
deltoideus medialis
vastus lateralis
deltoideus anterior
tibialis anterior
trapezius
coracobrachialis*
pectoralis minor*
rectus femoris
pectoralis major
vastus intermedius*
tensor fasciae latae
iliopsoas*
serratus anterior
transversus abdominis*
triceps brachii
rectus abdominis

Annotation Key
Bold text indicates target muscles
Black text indicates other working muscles
* indicates deep muscles

320 Swiss Ball Hand Walk-Around

Assume the Swiss Ball Shin Plank position (#319) and then lift, reach, and place your left hand to the side, followed by the right hand as you "walk" in a circle. Rotate 90 degrees to your left, or a quarter turn, and then hand walk back to the starting position. Repeat the entire sequence, moving to the right.

321 Swiss Ball Skier

Lie prone on a Swiss ball and move forward until your thighs are resting on the top of the ball. While maintaining your core position, rotate your trunk quickly to the left so that your legs are stacked on top of each other. Return to the starting position and perform the same movement to the right.

322 Swiss Ball Hand Walkout

Lie prone on a Swiss ball with your hips over the center of the ball as you support your weight on your arms. Your hands should be directly below your shoulders. Lift, reach, and place your left hand forward and then your right, rolling the ball underneath you until it reaches your feet.

323 Swiss Ball Plank with In-Out

Assume the Swiss Ball Shin Plank position (#319), making sure that your body forms a straight line from head to toes. Extend your left leg to the side, down off the ball. Return your leg to the ball, and then repeat on the other side.

324

Side Plank

The Side Plank is a superb move to tone your midsection while shoring up the strength of your lower back. To get the most from this exercise, aim to hold it with flawless form for at least a minute, and then repeat it for three sets on both sides. Once you have mastered this strategy, add in one of its many variations to your core-training drills.

· Lie on your right side with one arm supporting your torso, aligning your wrist under your shoulder. Place your left arm on top of your left leg. Your legs should be squeezed strongly together in adduction, with your legs parallel and your feet flexed. Draw your navel toward your spine.

· Press into the palm of your right hand and lift your hips off the floor, creating a straight line between your heels and head.

· Slowly lower your hips, returning to the starting position. Repeat the sequence for the desired repetitions, keeping your legs tight and your buttocks squeezed. Repeat on the other side.

Correct form
Keep your core tight and braced.

Avoid
Don't let your hips sag.

deltoideus anterior

brachioradialis

obliquus internus*

sartorius

vastus medialis

pectoralis major

pectoralis minor

rectus abdominis

biceps brachii

obliquus externus

vastus lateralis

rectus femoris

tensor fasciae latae

adductor longus

gracilis*

gastrocnemius

tibialis anterior

soleus

quadratus lumborum*

gluteus medius*

gluteus maximus

semitendinosus

biceps femoris

semimembranosus

Annotation Key
Bold text indicates target muscles
Black text indicates other working muscles
* indicates deep muscles

325 Forearm Side Plank

Lie on your right side with your arm bent so that you are resting on your forearm and supporting your torso. Pressing your left forearm into the floor, raise your hips off the ground until your body forms a long, straight line. Slowly lower your hips, returning to the starting position. Repeat the sequence for the desired repetitions, keeping your legs tight and your buttocks squeezed. Repeat on the other side.

326 Forearm Side Plank with Hip Raise on Aerobic Step

With your feet propped on a step, perform a Forearm Side Plank (#325). Repeat on the other side.

327 Forearm Side Plank with Knee Tuck

Perform as you would a Forearm Side Plank (#325), and bend your top knee to a 90-desgree angle, lifting it toward your chest. Repeat on the other side.

328 Forearm Side Plank with Toe Touch

Perform as you would a Forearm Side Plank (#325), and then extend your bottom leg upward as you extend your top arm to touch your fingers to your toes. Repeat on the other side.

329 Side-Bend Lift

Lie on your right side with your right hand behind your head and extend your left arm along the side of your body. Keeping your feet together, lift both legs upward. Repeat on the other side.

330 Lying Abduction

Lie on your right side with your arm bent so that your are resting on your forearm, supporting your torso. Extend your left arm along the side of your body, holding a dumbbell in that hand. Maintaining the position of the rest of your body, smoothly raise your top leg. Lower to the starting position. Repeat for the desired repetitions, and then repeat on the other side.

331 Lying Abduction into Side Plank

Perform as you would a Lying Abduction (#330), but when you return to the starting position, lift your hips to move into the Forearm Side Plank (#325). Lower to the starting position. Repeat on the other side.

T-Stabilization

T-Stabilization is an advanced variation of a High Plank exercise that effectively targets your abdominal, hip, lower-back, and oblique muscles. It also helps you work on improving your balance and coordination.

- Assume the drop position with your arms extended to full lockout, your fingers facing forward, your legs outstretched, and your body weight supported on your toes.

- Turn your hips to one side, stacking one foot on top of the other and raising your top arm across your body until you are pointing toward the ceiling.

- Hold for the desired time, lower, and then repeat on the other side to complete one rep.

biceps brachii

pectoralis major

deltoideus anterior

serratus anterior

rectus abdominis

obliquus externus

obliquus internus *

transversus abdominis*

vastus lateralis

brachioradialis

brachialis

pectineus

sartorius

gracilis*

tensor fasciae latae

rectus femoris

adductor longus

vastus medialis

tibialis anterior

soleus

Annotation Key
Bold text indicates target muscles
Black text indicates other working muscles
* indicates deep muscles

deltoideus posterior

triceps brachii

latissimus dorsi

gluteus medius*

tractus iliotibialis

gluteus maximus

adductor magnus

biceps femoris

semitendinosus

semimembranosus

Correct form
Engage your core, keeping your body in one straight line.

Avoid
Avoid arching or bridging your back.

333 Suspended T-Stabilization

Loop a suspension band over a sturdy object. Facing away from the anchor point, place your feet in the loop, and assume the drop position. Perform as you would the T-Stabilization (#332). Repeat on the other side.

334 Kneeling Forearm T-Stabilization

Assume the Forearm Side Plank position (#325). Pressing your forearm into the floor, raise your hips until your body forms a long, straight line. Repeat on the other side.

335 T-Stabilization with Leg Raise

Assume the Forearm Side Plank position (#325). Raise your top leg toward the ceiling while extending your top arm to reach for your toes. Repeat on the other side.

336 Plank with Rotation

Assume the drop position with your hands slightly wider than shoulder-width apart and with both feet on one towel. Draw both knees upward while simultaneously rotating your hips and lower body until your ankles are rotated 90 degrees and both feet are stacked and pointing to one side. Extend your knees and hips, and rotate back. Repeat on the other side.

337 T-Stabilization Twist

Lie on your right side with your legs extended and pressed firmly together. Press your right hip into the floor. Position your right hand directly beneath your shoulder, and press your body upward until you form a straight line from shoulder to feet. Extend your left arm toward the ceiling, and then bring your left arm down and across your torso, rotating your upper body to the right. Return to the starting position, and then repeat on the other side.

338 T-Stabilization with Reach-Under

Assume the Forearm Side Plank position (#325), propped on your left arm. Pressing your left forearm into the floor, raise your hips until your body forms a long, straight line. Twist your upper torso toward the floor as you reach your right arm under your chest as far as you can stretch. Twist your upper torso back to the front as you extend your right arm toward the ceiling. Complete the desired repetitions, and then switch sides.

339

Kneeling Side Kick

To strengthen your glutes, the Kneeling Side Kick is a can't-miss exercise. It particularly targets the hard-to-work gluteus medius (the smallest of the gluteal muscles). Strong glutes are essential for balanced movement during high-intensity workouts.

gluteus medius*
gluteus maximus
adductor magnus
biceps femoris
semitendinosus
semimembranosus

- Kneel with your right hand on the floor directly below your shoulder, with the fingers pointing outward. Place your left hand behind your head.

- Lift your left leg to hip level and straighten it. Keep your whole body aligned in one plane so that there is no rotation at the hips.

- Kick your left leg straight out in front of you, flexing your foot and trying not to move at your waist.

- Pull your left leg behind you, pointing your toes and keeping your leg at hip level. Repeat the sequence for the desired reps, and then repeat with the other leg.

rectus abdominis

obliquus externus

Correct form
Keep your torso and pelvis stable as you move your leg back and forth.

Avoid
Avoid wobbling as you kick—instead, make the movement smaller.

tensor fasciae latae

vastus lateralis

obliquus internus*

transversus abdominis*

rectus femoris

sartorius

iliopsoas*

pectineus*

adductor longus

gracilis*

vastus medialis

340 Swiss Ball Kneeling Side Lift

Prop your right arm on top of a Swiss ball and place your left hand on your hip. Begin leaning your torso to the right, and then lift your left leg as high as you can while keeping it in line with your hips. Kick your left leg straight out in front of you, flexing your foot and trying not to move at your waist. Pull your left leg behind you, pointing your toes and keeping your leg at hip height. Repeat the sequence for the desired reps, and then repeat with the other leg.

341 Kneeling Side Raise

Kneel on the floor and balance on your left knee with your left hand on the floor directly under your shoulder. Extend your right leg out to the side with your toes touching the floor and your right fingertips behind your head. Keeping your right leg straight, kick it forward at hip height. Flex your right foot and hold it for a second. Repeat the sequence for the desired reps, and then repeat with the other leg.

342 Kneeling Side Circles

Kneel on the floor with your right leg outstretched to the side and your left leg lined up under your hips. Place your left palm or fingertips on the floor and arch your right arm over your head. Lift your right leg and begin making small circles, gradually increasing to larger, sweeping circles. Perform the desired reps, switch sides, and repeat on the other leg.

343 Kneeling Side Lift

Kneel on the floor with your right leg outstretched to the side and your left leg lined up under your hips. Place both hands behind your head with your elbows extended out to the sides. Begin leaning your torso to the left, and then lift your right leg as high as you can while keeping it in line with your hips. Perform the desired reps, then switch sides and repeat on the other leg.

344

Swiss Ball Pike

Correct form
Position your hands so that they are directly below your shoulders.

Avoid
Don't allow your middle back to sag.

Swiss Ball Pike is a demanding exercise—it requires balance, stability, and precision to complete with accuracy and proper form. It is a particularly effective core-strengthener that works the rectus abdominis, and it also targets your hip flexors, external obliques, and spinal erectors. In the starting position, your sense of balance comes into play, and as you raise your hips, the strength of your core muscles is greatly challenged. For best results, concentrate on keeping your movement smooth.

· With a Swiss ball behind you, assume a drop position with your arms shoulder-width apart and your shins and the tops of your feet resting on the ball.

· While keeping your legs straight, roll the ball toward your body while raising your hips as high as you are able. Lower and repeat for the desired repetitions.

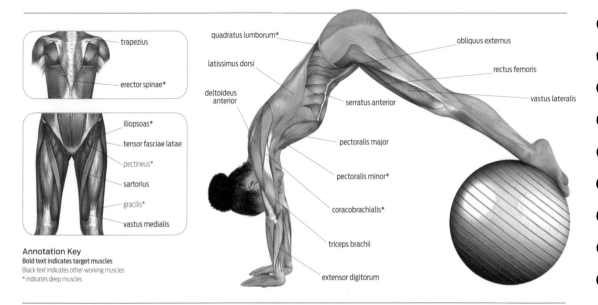

trapezius

erector spinae*

iliopsoas*

tensor fasciae latae

pectineus*

sartorius

gracilis*

vastus medialis

quadratus lumborum*

latissimus dorsi

deltoideus anterior

serratus anterior

obliquus externus

rectus femoris

vastus lateralis

pectoralis major

pectoralis minor*

coracobrachialis*

triceps brachii

extensor digitorum

Annotation Key
Bold text indicates target muscles
Black text indicates other working muscles
* indicates deep muscles

345 Pike

Start in a high plank position with the front of your body facing the floor in one long line and your weight on the balls of your feet. Keep your hands and feet solidly planted into the floor as you lift your hips toward the ceiling. Inhale in this inverted V position, extending your heels downward as you stretch your torso, arms, and legs downward into your mat. Exhale as you return to the high plank position. Repeat for the desired repetitions and sets.

346 Medicine Ball Pike

Assume a drop position with your hands shoulder-width apart and your toes planted on a Medicine ball. Raise your hips to the ceiling, rolling the Medicine ball toward your hands as you do so. Reverse the movement, lowering yourself back to the starting position. Repeat for the desired repetitions and sets.

347 Swiss Ball Pike and Press

Assume a drop position with your hands wider than shoulder-width apart on some blocks (or a bench) and plant your toes on a Swiss ball. Raise your hips to the ceiling, rolling the ball toward your hands as you do so. Keeping your torso in that position, bend your elbows and drop your spine head-first between your hands. Return by pushing your hands into the blocks until your elbows are fully extended. Then, drop your hips and extend your toes until your body returns to horizontal. Repeat for the desired repetitions and sets.

348 Swiss Ball Jackknife

Assume a push-up position with your arms shoulder-width apart and your shins resting on a Swiss ball. Bend your knees, rolling the ball in toward your chest, keeping your arms straight the whole time. Extend your legs, and repeat for the desired repetitions and sets.

349 Suspended Pike

Loop a suspension band over a sturdy object. Kneel facing away from the anchor point and place both feet in the loop of the band and plant your hands under your shoulders. Lift your knees off the ground into a plank position and raise your hips, keeping your legs straight. Lower your body back to plank position. Repeat for the desired repetitions and sets.

350

Plow

Known as Halasana in yoga, the Plow gets its name from the farming tool. It is an inverted forward-bending pose that challenges your flexibility and coordination. It also offers a thorough stretch for your shoulders and spine.

gluteus maximus · gluteus medius*
transversus abdominis* · obliquus internus*
biceps femoris · obliquus externus
· rectus abdominis
erector spinae* · latissimus dorsi
subscapularis* · triceps brachii
supraspinatus* · infraspinatus*

Annotation Key
Bold text indicates target muscles
Black text indicates other working muscles
* indicates deep muscles

Correct form
If the position feels hard on your neck, use a rolled-up blanket, foam pad, or cushion to protect your vertebrae.

Avoid
Avoid excessive speed, shallow or bouncy repetitions, or allowing your lower back to dip too far.

· Lie supine on the floor with your knees bent and your arms by your sides with your hands placed flat on the floor.

· Tighten your abdominals and lift your knees off the floor. Exhale, press your arms into the floor, and lift your knees higher so that your buttocks and hips come off the floor.

· Continue lifting your knees toward your face and roll your back off the mat from your hips to your shoulders. With your upper arms firmly planted on the floor, bend your elbows and place your hands on your lower back. Draw your elbows in closer to your sides.

· Inhale, tuck your tailbone toward your pubis, and straighten your legs back toward your head until your torso is perpendicular to the floor.

· Exhale and continue to extend your legs beyond your head. Squeeze your legs and bend at your waist until your toes touch the floor. Place your palms on the floor, pushing through your arms to maintain the lift in your hips. Hold for the desired time, and repeat.

351 Plow with Swiss Ball Adduction

Lie supine on the floor with your knees bent and your arms by your sides. Place your hands flat on the floor and grasp a Swiss ball between your feet. Perform as you would the Plow exercise (#350).

352 Swiss Ball Plow

Lie supine on the floor with your knees bent over a Swiss Ball, and then perform as you would the Plow exercise (#350).

Exercise Mats

Many exercises call for you to lie, sit, or kneel on the floor, which can be hard on your spine or joints. To protect your back and knees, working out on a mat makes sense. Keep in mind, though, that not all mats are the same. There are three basic varieties: yoga mats, fitness mats, and Pilates mats. Yoga mats, often called sticky mats, tend to be the thinnest—about a quarter to one inch (.6 to 2.5 cm) thick—and offer an nonslip surface that allows you to move from pose to pose without sliding. General-purpose fitness mats are thicker—up to three inches (7.5 cm)—and have more spring, which will help prevent falls and injuries while cushioning your back or joints. Pilates mats, like yoga mats, are sticky, but they are much thicker than yoga mats. The extra padding is essential, as so many Pilates exercises are performed lying on your back, sides, or stomach. This cushioning will protect you while you roll and rock.

353

Bridge

The Bridge exercise functions as a core strengthener, a back bend, and enhances core stability. It is a great way to efficiently target your glutes and hamstrings. To perform the Bridge exercise correctly, you need to keep your body in proper alignment—you want to form a straight line from your shoulders to your knees. If you feel yourself sagging, lower to the starting position, and then try again.

Correct form
To fully engage your core, try to pull your navel back toward your spine.

Avoid
Don't let your hips sag.

- Lie on your back with your legs bent, your feet flat on the floor, and your arms extended on the floor parallel to your body.

- Push through your heels while raising your pelvis until your torso is aligned with your thighs. Hold for the desired time, and then lower yourself back down.

vastus lateralis

rectus femoris

tensor fasciae latae

transversus abdominis*

Annotation Key
Bold text indicates target muscles
Black text indicates other working muscles
* indicates deep muscles

biceps femoris

obliquus externus

rectus abdominis

gastrocnemius

obliquus internus*

gluteus maximus

gluteus minimus*

gluteus medius*

triceps brachii

deltoideus medialis

354 Piriformis Bridge

Lie on your back with your arms extended at your sides and your knees with your feet flat on the floor. Keeping the rest of your body still, raise your left leg to rest the ankle on your right knee. Press your palms into the floor and engage your abdominal muscles as you lift. Your body should form a diagonal line from shoulders to knees. Slowly and with control, return to the starting position. Switch legs and repeat for the desired repetitions.

355 Bridge with High Knees

Perform the Bridge (#353), and then, keeping your legs bent, draw your left knee back, bringing it as close to your chest as possible. Lower your left leg until your toe touches the floor. Be sure to keep your pelvis level. Bring your left knee toward your chest again. Repeat the sequence for the desired repetitions, and then lower your left leg to the floor, and perform the exercise with your right leg. Repeat for the desired repetitions.

356 Bridge with Leg Lift

Perform the Bridge (#353), and then, keeping one knee bent, extend the other straight to the ceiling. Hold and then lower. Repeat the sequence for the desired repetitions, and then lower your leg to the floor, and perform the exercise with your other leg. Repeat for the desired repetitions.

357 Aerobic Step Bridge with Leg Lift and Chest Press

Holding a dumbbell or hand weight in each hand at chest level, lie on your back with your heels propped on an aerobic step and your knees bent. Extend one leg toward the ceiling. Push through the heel on the step as you raise your pelvis until your torso is aligned with your thighs, while at the same time pressing the weights straight up. Lower to the starting position, then repeat with the other leg. Repeat for the desired repetitions.

358 Suspended Bridge

Loop two suspension bands over a sturdy object. Facing the anchor point, place your feet in the loops and lie supine. Perform as you would the Bridge (#353). Repeat for the desired repetitions.

359
Roller Bridge with Leg Lift
Lie on your back with a roller under your feet. Without moving the roller or arching your back, bridge up and lift your hips into the air. Keeping your muscles firm, raise your right leg up to the height of your knees, then straighten your raised leg. Try to keep the roller from moving, and raise and lower your hips while keeping your outstretched leg raised. Repeat for the desired reps, and then switch legs.

360
Roller Bridge with Hamstring Pull-In
Lie supine on the floor, your knees bent and a foam roller under your feet. Perform as you would the Bridge (#353), lifting your hips so that they align with your shoulders in a neutral position. Squeeze your glutes and pull your calves in and out as you roll the roller under your feet. Repeat for the desired repetitions.

361
Roller Bridge with Leg Extension
Lie on your back with a roller under your shoulders. Your butt should be on the floor, with your knees bent and your feet flat on the floor. Press into the floor with your feet and bridge up, lifting your hips toward the ceiling until they are parallel to the floor. Extend your right leg and then raise it up to the height of your knees. Keeping your leg straight and the roller still, raise and lower your hips. Return to the Bridge position (#353), and then repeat with the left leg.

362

Swiss Ball Bridge

For many abdominal exercises, it is not the extent of your movements but the quality of them that makes the difference between an exercise that is effective and one that misses the target. The Swiss Ball Bridge is a perfect example—it is a powerful core exercise that also activates your glutes, lower back, and obliques.

Correct form
Contract your glutes and hold your stomach tight to keep your hips and shoulders parallel to the floor. To maintain your upper-body form, you can hold a pole or broomstick with your arms outspread.

Avoid
Don't allow your body to drop out of alignment: you should form a straight line from head to knees.

- Sit on the floor with your back against a Swiss ball. Bend your knees to 90 degrees and spread your arms wide at shoulder height.

- Push through your heels, and, using your glutes and hamstrings, raise your hips upward as you roll your back up the ball until your torso is aligned with your thighs.

- Hold the position for the desired time, and then lower yourself back down.

transversus abdominis* rectus abdominis adductor magnus

adductor longus

obliquus externus

adductor brevis

obliquus internus*

sartorius

iliopsoas*

tensor fasciae latae

rectus femoris

vastus intermedius*

Annotation Key
Bold text indicates target muscles
Black text indicates other working muscles
* indicates deep muscles

vastus lateralis

363

Backward Ball Stretch

The Backward Ball Stretch is a challenging flexibility exercise that targets your thoracic and upper-lumbar spine, along with your core muscles. It will help you increase spinal extension, while stretching your abs and latissimus dorsi muscles—the broad, flat muscles that cover much of your back on either side. It also helps you to develop balance and coordination.

- Sit on a Swiss ball in a well-balanced, neutral position, with your hips directly over the center of the ball.

- Raise your arms while maintaining good balance, and begin to extend them behind you.

- As you continue to extend your hands backward, walk your feet forward, allowing the ball to roll up your spine.

- As your hands touch the floor, extend your legs as far forward as you comfortably can. Hold this position for a few seconds.

- To deepen the stretch, extend your arms and walk your legs and hands closer to the ball. Hold this position for a few seconds.

- To release the stretch, bend your knees, drop your hips to the floor, lift your head off the ball, and then walk back to the starting position.

trapezius

latissimus dorsi

quadratus lumborum*

gluteus medius*

quadratus femoris*

Annotation Key
Bold text indicates target muscles
Black text indicates other working muscles
* indicates deep muscles

Correct form
Maintain good balance throughout the stretch. Move slowly and in a controlled manner. Keep your head on the ball until you have dropped your knees all the way down as you release from the stretch.

Avoid
Avoid any lateral ball movement, and do not hold the extended position for too long or until you feel dizzy.

rectus femoris

transversus abdominis*

rectus abdominis

serratus anterior

vastus lateralis

pectoralis major

pectoralis minor*

obliquus externus

deltoideus medialis

biceps femoris

biceps brachii

flexor carpi radialis

364 Backward Ball Stretch II

Perform as you would the Backward Ball Stretch (#363), but rather than extend your hands to the floor, roll only to your middle back and clasp your hands behind your head.

365 Swiss Ball Bridge with Rotation

Lie on a Swiss ball so that your upper back is on the ball with your hips unsupported. Plant your feet flat on the floor, hip-width apart or wider, and bend your knees to 90 degrees. Grasp a weighted ball with both hands and position your arms straight up. Rotate your upper body to the left, rolling onto your left shoulder on top of the Swiss ball. Hold briefly and then slowly roll back to the starting position with the Swiss ball in the center of your shoulders. Repeat the exercise, rotating your torso and rolling your shoulders to the right. Continue rotating from side to side for the desired time or repetitions.

366 Swiss Ball Bridge Side-to-Side Roll

Lie with your lower back on a Swiss ball with your feet together and your knees bent at 90 degrees. Position your arms out to the sides. Move your upper body across the ball to the left, rolling the ball under your shoulders and toward your left shoulder. Hold for five seconds and then slowly roll the ball back to the center of your shoulders. Return to the starting position, then roll to the right.

367 Standing Backbend

Stand tall with your feet placed at a comfortable width apart, your toes pointed forward or angled to the sides. Place your arms over your head, making sure that they are straight and tight with your hands flat, palms up, and fingers pointing behind you. Slowly arch backward and look downward for the floor. Keep your arms locked as you move closer to the floor. Place your hands on the floor, and keep your feet firmly planted. Your head should look back toward the floor while you hold the position.

Swiss Ball Leg Bridge

Annotation Key
Bold text indicates target muscles
Black text indicates other working muscles
* indicates deep muscles

The Swiss Ball Leg Bridge is low-intensity move that packs a lot of punch, effectively toning and strengthening your abdominals and glutes. You can amp up this basic move by adding leg lifts and curls to further increase its benefits.

erector spinae *

gluteus medius*

gluteus minimus*

gluteus maximus

adductor magnus

semitendinosus

semimembranosus

· Lie face-up on the floor with your arms at your sides and your lower legs resting on the Swiss ball.

· Press your palms into the floor and engage your abdominal muscles as you lift your upper body off the floor. Your body should form a diagonal line. If desired, hold for a few seconds.

· Slowly and with control, lower down to the starting position. Repeat for the desired repetitions.

Correct form
Fully engage your abs to keep your body in a stable line from feet to shoulders.

Avoid
Don't allow your hips to sag.

rectus abdominis

quadratus lumborum*

biceps femoris

gluteus maximus

gastrocnemius

369 Swiss Ball Bridge with Leg Raises

Perform as you would the Swiss Ball Leg Bridge (#368), and then in the raised position, lift one leg off the ball, extending it upward while maintaining your form. Return to the starting position. Repeat on the other side, keeping both legs straight and your back neutral as you move. Continue for the desired repetitions.

370 Swiss Ball Bridge with Leg Curl

Lie on the floor with your arms out to the sides at shoulder height or extended along your sides, palms down, and perform as you would the Swiss Ball Leg Bridge (#368). From the raised position, pull your heels toward you and roll the ball as close to your butt as possible. Pause, then roll back to the Bridge position, lower your hips to the floor, and continue for the desired repetitions.

371

Bird Dog

High-intensity workouts can be hard on your lower back, so including exercises that support the muscles of your spine—especially the lumbar region—can help you stave off discomfort and keep you ready to work hard. The Bird Dog, also called the Quadruped Arm/Leg Raise, targets a group of deep muscles that run along your spinal column called the erector spinae muscles, which work to extend your torso. As well as being an effective lower-back move, the Bird Dog is a classic that will help you hone your balance, stability, and coordination.

Correct form
Your movements show be controlled and steady to decrease pelvic rotation.

Avoid
Avoid tilting your pelvis during the movement—slide your leg along the surface of the mat before lifting. Don't allow your back to sink into an arched position.

· Kneel on all fours with your hands under your shoulders and your knees under your hips, while keeping your head, neck, and back straight. Engage your abdominals by drawing your navel up toward your spine.

· Raise your right arm and reach it forward until it is in line with your torso. At the same time, kick your left leg upward until it is parallel to the floor, while keeping your torso still.

· Bring your arm and leg back to the starting position, then repeat the sequence on the other side, alternating for the desired time or repetitions.

Annotation Key
Bold text indicates target muscles
Black text indicates other working muscles
* indicates deep muscles

gluteus medius*

transversus abdominis*

obliquus externus

gluteus maximus

biceps femoris

rectus femoris

deltoideus medialis

adductor magnus

rectus abdominis

adductor longus

tensor fasciae latae

obliquus internus*

372 Pointer

Assume the drop position, and then extend your left arm straight forward while raising your right leg until your body forms a straight line from toe to shoulder. Pause at the top of the movement, and then lower back to the drop position. Repeat on the opposite side.

373 Foam Roller Quadruped Knee Pull-In

Challenge your balance as well as your core strength and stability with the Foam Roller Quadruped Knee Pull-In. This exercise also helps to strengthen your shoulders, which will help prepare you for vigorous high-intensity throwing exercises.

- Place a foam roller on the floor and kneel on it with your hands placed on the floor in front of you. Your hands should be slightly in front of your torso, and your hips should be lifted off your heels.

- Round out your torso as you pull your knees toward your hands, allowing the roller to move toward your feet. Repeat for the desired reps and sets.

Foam Rollers

Foam rollers are useful tools in a fitness kit. Like Swiss balls and balance ball trainers, they can add an element of instability to an exercise, which can help you hone your balance, improve your strength, and increase your cardio endurance. Performing basic exercises, like Push-Ups, Squats, and Planks, on the unstable surface of a roller boosts the challenge to the targeted muscles. Foam rollers, which are simply dense foam cylinders (either smooth or knobbly), are relatively inexpensive and highly portable. As well as using them for strength and cardio exercises, you can use them for self-myofascial release (SMFR). To use it properly for SMFR, you need to control your body weight on the foam roller to generate the pressure necessary to break up problematic spots, known as trigger points. This effective form of self-massage is a great way to relieve soreness after a vigorous, high-intensity interval workout.

374

Fire Hydrant

The Fire Hydrant exercise, also known as the Quadruped Left Lift, is a multifaceted move that targets your core muscles, pelvic stabilizers, and abductor leg muscles. It can improve your pelvic stability and strengthen your hips and legs.

· Kneel on your hands and knees, your spine in neutral position.

· Keep your weight centered and raise your right knee—still bent—out to the side.

· Raise and lower your leg without moving your hips. Repeat for the desired reps, and then switch legs.

Correct form
Maintain a neutral spine to prevent your lower back from sagging. Keep your chin tucked in, and press your hands into the floor to keep your shoulders from sinking near your ears.

Avoid
Avoid lifting your hip as you lift your leg.

Annotation Key
Bold text indicates target muscles
Black text indicates other working muscles
* indicates deep muscles

gluteus medius*

transversus abdominis*

obliquus externus

gluteus maximus

tractus iliotibialis

rectus abdominis

vastus intermedius*

vastus lateralis

obliquus internus*

adductor magnus

sartorius

rectus femoris

vastus medialis

gracilis*

375 Straight-Leg Fire Hydrant

Kneel on your hands and knees, then lift one leg straight up until it is parallel to the floor, making sure to keep it in line with your hip. Return to the starting position and repeat with the opposite leg. Continue to alternate for the desired repetitions.

376 Fire Hydrant In-Out

Kneel on your hands and knees, resting your right arm on your forearm, palms down, and lining up your left arm under your shoulder. Your spine should be in a neutral position. Keeping your left leg bent at a 90-degree angle, raise it to the side and then straighten it until it is fully extended behind you so that it is in line with your torso. Continue for the desired repetitions, and then repeat on the other side.

377 Clamshell Series

The Clamshell Series takes you through a sequence of movements that will work both your inner and outer thighs while challenging your coordination.

· Lie on your right side with your knees bent and stacked on top of each other. Bend your left elbow, placing it directly underneath your shoulder so that your forearm is supporting your upper body. Place your left hand on your hip.

· Without moving your hips, open your left knee upward and then return to the starting position. Repeat for the desired repetitions.

· Lift both ankles off the floor, making sure to maintain a straight line with the torso.

· While your ankles are still lifted, lift and lower your left knee to open and close your legs. Repeat for the desired repetitions.

· The final part of this series begins with both ankles elevated. Lift your left knee to separate your legs, and then straighten your left leg, being careful not to move the position of your thigh. Bend your knee and return to the starting position. Repeat for the desired repetitions, and then repeat all steps on the opposite side.

378

Squat Thrust

The Squat Thrust is a powerhouse of an exercise, combining the strength-training benefits of a squat or push-up move with high-intensity cardio. On its own, this exercise is challenging, but it is also the main component of the classic Burpee.

- Stand with your feet hip-width apart and your arms above your head.

- Drop into a squat position, and then place your hands on the floor.

- In one quick, explosive motion, kick your feet back to assume a drop position.

- In another quick motion, push through both feet to return to the squat position.

- Continue performing for the desired time or repetitions.

erector spinae*

deltoideus posterior

serratus anterior

gluteus medius*

deltoideus anterior

tensor fasciae latae

vastus medialis

gluteus maximus

vastus intermedius*

brachialis

biceps femoris

Correct form
Keep your core tight and braced.

semitendinosus

rectus femoris

Avoid
Don't let your hips sag. Make sure you keep your back flat as you perform the drop position portion of this exercise.

semimembranosus

vastus lateralis

gastrocnemius

Annotation Key
Bold text indicates target muscles
Black text indicates other working muscles
* indicates deep muscles

tibialis anterior

soleus

379 Dumbbell Squat Thrust

Stand with your feet shoulder-width apart, holding a dumbbell in each hand. Perform as you would a Squat Thrust (#378). Repeat for the desired time or repetitions.

380 Burpee

The names Burpee and Squat Thrust are often used interchangeably, but there is an important difference: a Burpee takes you through the same moves as a Squat Thrust but adds a jump at the end. This plyometric boost takes this already powerful calisthenic exercise to the next level, amping up its cardio and strength benefits. Challenge yourself with one of this versatile exercise's many variations; for example, you can add different kinds of jumps or perform it on one leg.

· Stand with your feet hip-width apart and your arms above your head.

· Drop into a squat position, placing your hands on the floor.

· In one quick, explosive motion, kick your feet back to assume a drop position to perform a Basic Push-Up (#226).

· In another quick motion, jump into the air, and return to the starting position. Continue performing for the desired time or repetitions.

381 Burpee with Pull-Up

Stand with your shoulders positioned under a pull-up bar. Perform a Burpee (#380), and then return to the drop position. From there, jump up to reach for the bar with your arms fully extended, grasping the bar with an overhand grip. In a smooth motion, pull your body up and then lower it until your arms are again fully extended. Return to the standing position, and then continue performing all steps for the desired time or repetitions.

382 Side Burpee

Perform as you would a Burpee (#380), but instead of jumping your feet straight out into the drop position, jump your legs out to the side so your body is at a diagonal. Alternate jumping to the right and left as you continue for the desired time or repetitions.

383 Renegade Burpee

Stand with your feet hip-width apart, holding a kettlebell or dumbbell in each hand. Drop into a squat position, and place the weights on the floor. Kick your feet back into the drop position with your hands still on top of the weights and shoulder-width apart. Holding the drop position, bend your right elbow and raise the dumbbell until your elbow passes your torso while pressing into your left arm for balance. Lower your right arm and perform the same row action with your left arm. Return your feet back to the squat position, under your hips, and then stand up. Alternate right and left rows as you continue for the desired time or repetitions.

384 Burpee with Push-Up to Clap

Perform as you would a Burpee (#380), and then from the Push-Up, explode upward and clap your hands. Land with soft, bent elbows, and then continue for the desired time or repetitions.

385 Tuck-Jump Burpee

Stand with your feet hip-width apart and your arms above your head or extended at your sides. Drop into a squat position, placing your hands on the floor. In one quick, explosive motion, kick your feet back to assume a drop position to perform a Basic Push-Up (#226). Hop your feet back into a squat, and then jump explosively upward, tucking your knees tight into your chest. Land softly on the balls of your feet to return to the starting position. Repeat for the desired time or repetitions.

386 Box-Jump Burpee

Stand in front of a high aerobic step or low box. Perform as you would a Burpee (#380), but jump up onto the step when you come up rather than jumping straight up in place. Continue for the desired time or repetitions.

387 Burpee Broad Jump

Assume a squat position with your heels outside of your shoulders and your toes slightly pointed outward. Propel yourself into a jump off both feet, jumping as far forward as far as possible. As you land, bend your hips and knees while leaning forward until your hands touch the floor. Immediately jump both feet backward into the drop position. From the drop position, reverse the process.

388 Single-Leg Burpee

Stand with your weight entirely on one leg and bend your opposite knee to lift your foot from the floor. Bend your standing leg and squat, placing your hands on the floor under your shoulders. Jump your leg behind you to bring your body into a straight line, then immediately hop it back towards your hands and explode upwards into the air. Continue, switching legs with each repetition.

389 Single-Arm Burpee

Stand with your feet slightly wider than hip-width apart and your left arm out to the side at shoulder height. Squat down, and place your right hand on the floor, just under the center of your chest. Tighten your abs and jump your feet back into a one-arm plank. Quickly jump back toward your hands, landing in a squat. Repeat for the desired time or repetitions.

390 Burpee Deck Squats

Place a mat on the floor and stand in front of it with your back to it. Squat down to your toes, roll back on the mat bringing your legs as far back as you can, and then roll back up. As soon as you stand up, perform a Burpee (#380). Repeat for the desired time or repetitions.

391

Scissors

The Scissors exercise, taken from the demanding discipline of Pilates, improves core stability and increases abdominal strength and endurance. It can be modified by performing all the repetitions on one leg before switching to the other.

- Lie supine on the floor or a mat, your arms by your sides and your legs raised in a tabletop position. Inhale, drawing in your abdominals.

- Stretching your right leg away from your body, raise your left leg toward your trunk. Hold your left calf with your hands, pulsing twice while keeping your shoulders down.

- Switch your legs in the air, reaching for your right leg. Stabilize your pelvis and spine. Repeat the sequence for the desired repetitions on each leg.

Annotation Key
Bold text indicates target muscles
Black text indicates other working muscles
* indicates deep muscles

biceps femoris

flexor digitorum

rectus abdominis

brachioradialis

transversus abdominis*

brachialis

rectus femoris

vastus lateralis

iliopsoas*

obliquus externus

triceps brachii

deltoideus medialis

392 Single-Leg Circles

Lie flat on the floor with both legs and arms extended. Bend your right knee toward your chest and then straighten your leg upward. Anchor the rest of your body to the floor, straightening both knees and pressing your shoulders back and down. Cross your raised leg up and over your body, aiming for your left shoulder. Continue making a circle with the raised leg, returning to the center. Switch directions so that you aim your leg away from your body. Repeat with the other leg.

393 Single-Leg Calf Press

Sit with your legs outstretched in front of you, with a foam roller placed under your ankles. Place your hands on the floor to support your torso, your fingers pointing forward. Press into the floor to lift your hips, keeping your legs firm. Lift one leg off the roller and hold it steady, making sure not to drop your hips. Keep your leg elevated and press your opposite leg into the roller, drawing your hips back toward your hands. Return to the starting position, rolling your calf muscle along the roller and keeping your lifted leg straight in the air. Repeat with the other leg.

394 Foam Roller Bicycle

Lie supine with a roller placed lengthwise under your spine, your buttocks and shoulders resting on the roller. Place your forearms on the floor on either side of the roller to balance yourself. Draw your knees up to a tabletop position, and then keeping your back flat, lift your head, neck, and shoulders off the roller. Straighten your right leg and pull your left knee toward your chest, keeping your head, neck, and shoulders lifted. Switch legs while maintaining your balance, imitating the pedaling of a bicycle. Repeat on the other side.

395 Abdominal Kicks

Lie in supine position with your legs extended. Lift from the shoulders as you pull your right knee toward your chest and straighten your left leg, raising it about 45 degrees from the floor. Place your right hand on your right ankle, and your left hand on your right knee. Keep switching your hand and leg placement for the desired repetitions.

396 Supine Marches

Lie lengthwise on a foam roller. Place your arms on the floor by your sides, bending your knees so that your feet rest flat on the floor. Pointing your toes and keeping your hips from lifting or shifting, raise one knee toward your chest, being careful to keep your hips stationary. Continue alternating legs as you establish a smooth "marching" rhythm.

397 Tiny Steps

Lie supine with your knees bent and feet flat on the floor. Place your hands on your hip bones. Raise your right knee to your chest while pulling your navel toward your spine. Hold the position at the top. As you continue to pull your navel toward your spine, lower your right leg onto the floor while controlling any movement in your hips. Alternate legs to complete the full movement. Continue for the desired repetitions.

398

Correct form
Keep your abs tight.

Avoid
Avoid allowing your lower back to lift.

Double Leg Raise

The Double Leg Raise looks like a simply move—and it is in theory. But in practice, this exercise presents a strong challenge to your abdominals and hip flexors. Mastering this intense Pilates staple can result in a strong, stable core.

· Lie on your back with your arms along your sides, and extend your legs straight up toward the ceiling. Rotate your legs out slightly, keeping the heels together, the inner legs pulled in the center line, and your toes pointed.

· Lower your legs so that your feet are just above the floor, and then raise them back to the starting position.

soleus
rectus femoris
transversus abdominis*
rectus abdominis
obliquus internus *
gastrocnemius
obliquus externus
semimembranosus
vastus lateralis
tensor fasciae latae

Annotation Key
Bold text indicates target muscles
Black text indicates other working muscles
* indicates deep muscles

399 Hip Twist

Begin by sitting on the floor with your arms behind your body, supporting your weight. Your legs should be parallel and raised to a high diagonal. Engage your abdominals and shoulders for stabilization. Start to bring both legs across your body to the right. Continue to circle your legs across your body and down as low as you can while maintaining pelvic stabilization. Return your legs to the starting position. Repeat for the desired reps in each direction.

400 Corkscrew

Lie supine with your arms along your sides, palms down. Imprint your spine and lengthen your legs— one at a time—to the ceiling. Keep your legs parallel, firmly pressed together. Stabilize your shoulder blades and your pelvis against the weight of your legs as you inhale and begin circling your legs to the right and down. Continue to circle your legs as you complete the circle on an exhalation. Repeat, "drawing" a circle in the other direction.

401 Abdominal Hip Lift

Lie supine with your arms along your sides, palms down. Lift your legs straight in the air and cross them at the ankles. Pinching your legs together and squeezing your glutes, press into the back of your arms to lift your hips upward. Slowly return your hips to the floor. Perform for the desired reps, and then switch with the opposite leg crossed in the front.

402 Hip Lift with Arm Reach

Keeping your hips on the floor, raise your arms toward the ceiling. Reach toward your toes as you lift your shoulders off the floor.

403

Tabletop Ab Press

The Tabletop Ab Press, also known as the 90-Degree Static Press, demonstrates how an isometric, static exercise can reap high-intensity benefits. It effectively engages your core, and it will also get these muscles ready for a high-energy workout. Its tabletop position is also the base for other dynamic exercises.

Correct form
To fully engage your core, imagine that you are "zipping" your muscles from your pelvic floor up to your navel.

Avoid
Avoid lifting your shoulders from the floor.

vastus lateralis

rectus femoris

biceps femoris

vastus intermedius*

obliquus externus

biceps brachii

tensor fasciae latae

quadratus lumborum*

gluteus maximus

deltoideus posterior

triceps brachii

iliopsoas*

gluteus medius*

- Lie on your back with your knees and feet lifted, your thighs making a 90-degree angle with your upper body. This is the tabletop position.

- Place your hands on the front of your knees with your fingers facing upward, one palm on each leg.

- Flex your feet and, keeping your elbows bent and pulled into your sides, press your hands into your knees. Create resistance by pushing back against your hands with your knees. Hold for up to a minute, and then repeat for the desired repetitions.

rectus abdominis

transversus abdominis*

pectineus*

sartorius

Annotation Key
Bold text indicates target muscles
Black text indicates other working muscles
* indicates deep muscles

404 Dead Bug

Lie supine with a foam roller placed lengthwise under your spine, your buttocks and shoulders resting on the roller. Place your hands and forearms flat on the floor for stabilization. Draw your knees up so that your legs form a tabletop position. Lift your head, neck, and shoulders. Press the palms of your hands onto your knees, creating your own resistance as you try to balance. Flex your toes and keep your elbows pulled in to your sides. Hold for a few seconds, release, and then repeat for the desired repetitions.

405 Swiss Ball Tabletop Rotation

Lie supine in tabletop position with a Swiss ball between your knees. Press your shoulder blades into the floor, and move your legs and the Swiss ball toward your left. Your hips should roll along with your body, but try to keep the rest of your torso on the floor. Return to the starting position, and then bring the ball toward the left. Continue to alternate sides for the desired repetitions.

406 Hip Crossover

Lie supine with your knees and feet lifted in tabletop position, your thighs making a 90-degree angle with your upper body. Brace your abdominals and lower your legs to one side, as close to the floor as you can possibly go without raising your shoulders off the floor. Return to the starting position and then repeat on the other side. Continue to alternate sides for the desired repetitions.

407 Swiss Ball Hip Crossover

Lie on your back with your arms extended out to your sides. Place your legs on a Swiss ball, with your glutes close to the ball so that your lower body assumes the tabletop position. Perform as you would the Hip Crossover (#406). Continue to alternate sides for the desired repetitions.

408

Half Curl-Up

Correct form
Keep your arms parallel to the floor throughout the exercise.

Avoid
Avoid curling your neck too far forward or allowing your feet to lift off the floor.

The Half Curl-Up is a simple upper-abdominal exercise that strengthens your core muscles, protecting your back while increasing muscle tone.

· Lie on your back with your knees bent and arms straight by your sides. Squeeze your legs together and keep your feet flat on the floor.

· Using your upper abdominals, curl your upper back and shoulders upward so that your middle back remains pressed to the floor. Keep your arms parallel to the floor and your lower back flat.

· Hold for a few seconds and then return to the starting position. Repeat for the desired repetitions.

Annotation Key
Bold text indicates target muscles
Black text indicates other working muscles
* indicates deep muscles

rectus abdominis

deltoideus anterior

obliquus externus

pectoralis major

extensor digitorum

obliquus internus*

brachioradialis

biceps brachii

triceps brachii

sternocleidomastoideus

sternohyoideus

409 McGill Curl-Up

High-intensity interval training can be hard on your back, so incorporating certain moves into your regimen to protect it can help you prevent injury and discomfort. The McGill Curl-Up, also known as the McGill Crunch, may look like a simple move, but it is an effective exercise to strengthen both your core and your lumbar spine.

· Lie supine with your right leg fully extended and your left leg bent. Place both hands palm-down beneath your lower back.

· Keeping your abdominal muscles braced, contract them slightly, bringing your head and shoulders off the floor. Hold for a 5-second count.

· Lower your head, repeat for the desired repetitions, and then switch legs.

410 Curl-Up

Lie on your back with your knees bent and your arms straight by your sides. Squeeze your legs together and keep your feet flat on the floor. Using your upper abdominals, curl your upper back and shoulders upward until your middle back is fully lifted from the floor. Keep your arms parallel to the floor and your lower back flat and pressed into the floor. Hold for a few seconds, then return to the starting position. Repeat for the desired repetitions.

411 Tabletop Curl-Up

Lie on your back with your knees and feet lifted, your thighs making a 90-degree angle with your upper body to assume the tabletop position. Perform as you would the Curl-Up (#410). Repeat for the desired repetitions.

412 Swiss Ball Curl-Up

Lie on your back with your arms extended by your sides. Place your legs on a Swiss ball with your glutes close to the ball so that your lower body assumes the tabletop position. Perform as you would a Half Curl-Up (#408). Repeat for the desired repetitions.

413

Crunch

Long the go-to strength move for toning the abdominals, the Crunch has scores of variations, and many of them can be incorporated into a high-intensity regimen. Form is essential, so mastering the basics can help you work in its more demanding versions.

Correct form
Fully engage your abs; this tension will help ensure that you do not overarch your back.

Avoid
Avoid pulling on your neck or drawing your elbows in, which may strain your neck muscles and vertebrae.

Annotation Key
Bold text indicates target muscles
Black text indicates other working muscles
* indicates deep muscles

pectoralis major

serratus anterior

transversus abdominis*

obliquus externus

coracobrachialis*

serratus anterior

latissimus dorsi

tensor fasciae latae

iliopsoas*

· Lie supine on the floor with your knees bent and clasp your hands behind your head.

· Keeping your elbows wide, engage the abdominals and lift your upper torso to achieve a crunching movement.

· Return to the starting position. Continue at a quick but controlled pace.

414 Reverse Crunch

Lie supine on the floor and extend your arms at your sides. Raise your knees and feet so that they create a 90-degree angle. Contract your abdominals and exhale as you lift your hips off the floor; your knees will move toward your head. Inhale, then slowly lower.

415 Cable Crunch

Kneel in front of a cable station with a rope attachment connected to the top pulley. Grip the rope, resting your wrists against your forehead. Flex your hips slightly to take the weight and to hyperextend your lower back. Keeping your hips stationary, bend at the waist so that your elbows move down toward the middle of your thighs. Hold for one count, then return to the starting position.

416 Lemon Squeezer

Lie supine on the floor with your legs straight and your arms at your sides. Lift your legs, head, neck, and shoulders slightly off the floor and then raise your arms until they are parallel to the floor. Pulling your knees in toward your chest, reach your arms toward your ankles so that your torso lifts completely off the floor. Slowly open up, lengthening your legs and lowering back to the starting position. Repeat the motion without completely lying down. Repeat for the desired repetitions.

417 Standing Knee Crunch

Standing tall with your right leg in front of your left, extend your hands toward the ceiling, your arms straight. Shift your weight onto your right foot and raise your left knee to hip height. Simultaneously rise on the toes of your right foot while sharply pulling your elbows down by your sides to create the crunch. Pause at the top of the movement and then return to the starting position. Perform the sequence with your left leg as the standing leg. Repeat for the desired repetitions, alternating sides.

418 Punching Abs

Sit with your legs extended and feet together, knees slightly bent. Brace your core and lean back slightly with your fists at each side of your chest and your elbows bent. Punch your right fist forward at shoulder height, then quickly return to the starting position and repeat on the other side. Continue alternating punching right and left for the desired repetitions.

419 Forearm Side Plank Crunch

Get into the Forearm Side Plank position (#325). Bend your top elbow while at the same time bending your top knee and bringing it toward your elbow to create the crunch. Perform the desired repetitions, then repeat on the other side.

420 Foam Roller Diagonal Crunch

Lie lengthwise on a foam roller. With your legs straight and your feet pressed into the floor, extend your arms over your head. As you raise your head, neck, and shoulders, leave your right leg and left arm on the floor, using your hand for support. Raise your left leg and right arm and reach for your ankle. Return to the starting position and repeat on the other side.

421 Tabletop Crunch

Get into the tabletop position with your knees bent so that your shins are parallel to the floor, and then perform as you would a Crunch (#413). Repeat for the desired repetitions.

422 Swiss Ball Tabletop Crunch

Lie supine in the tabletop position with the back of your calves resting on a Swiss Ball. Perform as you would a Crunch (#413). Repeat for the desired repetitions.

423 Swiss Ball Crunch

Plant your feet firmly on the floor, and prop your back on a Swiss Ball with your head and neck supported, your legs bent, your palms placed on your ears, and your elbows flared outward. Raise your head and shoulders off the ball while contracting your torso toward your waist, keeping your lower back on the ball. Lower and repeat for the desired repetitions.

424 Chair Crunch

Sit on a chair with your hands grasping the sides of the seat and your arms straight. Step forward, bending your knees and lifting your butt off the chair. Your hips and knees should be bent to form 90-degree angles. Tuck your tailbone toward the front of the chair and bring your knees toward your chest. Bend your elbows simultaneously. At the bottom of the movement, extend your elbows and press through your shoulders. Keeping your head in neutral position, press into the chair and lower your legs to return to the starting position. Repeat for the desired repetitions.

425 L-Sit

Sit with your back straight and your legs straight in front of you, your hands placed next to your hips, palms down. Press strongly into the floor to push yourself up so that your butt and legs rise from the floor. Hold for the desired time period.

426 Kettlebell L-Sit

Sit with your legs straight in front of you, your hands grasping the handles of a kettlebell placed next to your hips. Perform as you would an L-Sit (#425). Hold for the desired time period. You can also perform this version on parallel bars.

427 Crossover Crunch

The Crossover Crunch adds a literal twist to the basic crunch, calling for a greater contribution from the oblique muscles that run along the side of your ribcage. It helps give you a total core workout and can also help stabilize your back—and a strong back is crucial for any high-intensity workout regimen.

- Bring your hands behind your head, lifting your legs off the floor into a tabletop position.

- Roll up with your torso, reaching your right elbow to your left knee and extending your right leg in front of you. Imagine pulling your shoulder blades off the floor and twisting from your ribs and oblique muscles. Continue to alternate sides in a quick but controlled pace.

428 Bent-Leg Crossover Crunch

Begin with both feet on the floor. Place the outside of one foot on top of your thigh near your knee. Perform as you would the Crossover Crunch (#427). Repeat for the desired repetitions.

429 Side Raised-Leg Crunch

Lie on your side with your legs slightly bent, your lower hand on your stomach and your upper hand behind your head. Raise your head and shoulders off the floor as you lift your legs, keeping your feet together. Lower and repeat for the desired repetitions, and then switch sides.

430 Penguin Crunch

Lie supine with your knees bent, your head elevated, and your arms straight at your sides and raised off the floor. Holding your torso in a flexed position, lean to the right and reach your right hand forward. Hold for one count and then pull it back. Repeat on your left side. Continue to alternate sides for the desired repetitions.

431 Alternating Crunch

Lie supine with your legs bent. Place your palms behind your ears, flaring your elbows outward. Raise your head and shoulders off the floor while contracting your trunk toward your waist as you rotate your elbow toward the opposite knee. Lower and repeat on the other side. Continue to alternate sides for the desired repetitions.

432 Straight-Leg Hanging Knee Raise

Grab a pull-up bar with your palms facing forward. Rise up on your toes and then lift your body so that your feet are not touching the ground. Pull on the bar so that your shoulders are down and away from your ears, keeping your legs straight and your knees and ankles taut. Keeping your lower back flat, kick forward to bring both legs up to horizontal. Slowly allow your legs to drop in a controlled manner until they are directly beneath you, back to the starting position. Repeat for the desired repetitions.

433 Bent-Knee Hanging Knee Raise with Weighted Ball

Hang with your upper arms cradled in ab straps attached to a pull-up bar, clasping a weighted ball between your knees. Grasp the top of the stirrups with your hands and pull your upper arms and elbows downward and your upper legs and knees upward toward your elbows, flexing at the hips. Return to the starting position in a slow and controlled manner. Repeat for the desired repetitions.

434 Hanging Knee Raise with Rotation

Hang with your upper arms cradled in ab straps attached to a pull-up bar. Keep your elbows bent at 90-degree angles, pointing forward just above shoulder height. Grasp the straps with your hands and pull your upper arms and elbows downward while rotating your upper legs and knees up toward your elbows, flexing at the hips. Tuck your hips forward and also bring your chest forward slightly. Return to the starting position in a slow and controlled manner. Repeat for the desired repetitions.

435 Layout on Straps

Attach suspension bands to a pull-up bar and place an aerobic step under the pull-up bar. Standing on the step with your body rigid at a 45-degree angle to the floor, grasp the bands directly under your shoulders with a palms-down grip. Your hands should be parallel and directly beneath your chest, with your legs, hips, and spine forming a straight line. With your arms straight, push your hands forward and outward, using your toes as a fulcrum and allowing your entire body to descend in a controlled manner until your arms are in a horizontal position. Return by pulling your arms back toward the floor until your body returns to the starting position. Repeat for the desired repetitions.

436

Turkish Get-Up

The Turkish Get-Up is a simple but comprehensive exercise that targets a wide range of muscles, including those in the shoulders, core, thighs, back, glutes, and arms. It increases stability in the hips and aids balance throughout the body. Make it more of a challenge by holding a dumbbell or kettlebell in your raised hand.

- Lie flat on your back. Raise your right arm straight out above your chest and extend your left arm along your side.

- Flex your right knee and place your right foot flat on the floor next to your left knee.

- Rotate your torso slightly to the left and lift your shoulders off the floor. Plant your left hand on the floor and lift yourself up to a sitting position.

- Lift your hips upward, and tuck your left leg under your body to support yourself on your left knee.

- Lift your left hand off the floor and push through your right foot to a standing position, keeping your right arm stretched over your head throughout the exercise.

- Return to the starting position. Perform for the desired repetitions and then repeat on the other side.

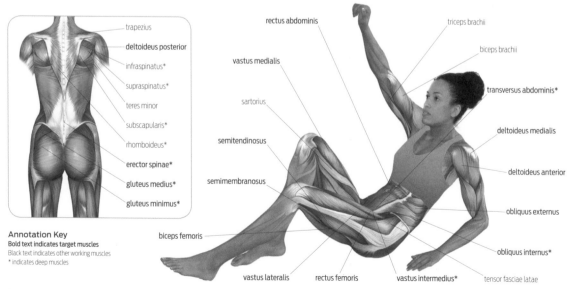

trapezius
deltoideus posterior
infraspinatus*
supraspinatus*
teres minor
subscapularis*
rhomboideus*
erector spinae*
gluteus medius*
gluteus minimus*

rectus abdominis
vastus medialis
sartorius
semitendinosus
semimembranosus
biceps femoris
vastus lateralis
rectus femoris

triceps brachii
biceps brachii
transversus abdominis*
deltoideus medialis
deltoideus anterior
obliquus externus
obliquus internus*
vastus intermedius*
tensor fasciae latae

Annotation Key
Bold text indicates target muscles
Black text indicates other working muscles
* indicates deep muscles

437

Sit-Up

The Sit-Up is to the abdominals what the bench press is to the pectorals: a highly effective exercise. The iconic Sit-Up is widely used on a daily basis and for good reason: it's the perfect exercise for the rectus abdominis. It is similar to a Crunch, but Sit-Ups have a fuller range of motion and condition additional muscles.

· Lie supine with your legs bent and your hands clasped behind your head.

· Start by pushing through your heels for support and raising your trunk off the ground, contracting your abdominals while lifting up toward your knees.

· Lower and repeat for the desired repetitions.

Annotation Key
Bold text indicates target muscles
Black text indicates other working muscles
* indicates deep muscles

coracobrachialis*

latissimus dorsi

obliquus externus

tensor fasciae latae

rectus abdominis

pectoralis major

serratus anterior

transversus abdominis*

iliopsoas*

438 Sit-Up and Throw

Lie supine with your legs bent and your feet firmly planted on the floor. Grasp a weighted ball and hold it behind your head with both hands. Bring your arms forward while rising off the ground and contracting your abdominals. Throw the ball to a partner. Receive it back, lower, and repeat.

439 Alternating Sit-Up

Lie supine with your legs slightly bent and your hands clasped behind your head. Push through your heels for support and raise your trunk off the floor. Rotate to the left so your elbow touches your opposite knee, and contract your abdominals. Lower and repeat, rotating to the other side. Continue alternating sides for the desired repetitions.

440

V-Up

The V-Up, also known as a Pike Crunch or Jackknife, is a challenging core movement. It has multiple benefits, including strengthening your abdominal muscles and increasing your overall flexibility and coordination. Performing V-Ups is also an efficient way to strengthen your lower-back muscles and tighten your quadriceps.

- Lie on your back with your legs extended and your arms raised overhead, your palms facing each other.

- Raise your legs to an angle between 45 and 90 degrees and then inhale, reaching your arms toward the ceiling as you lift your head and shoulders off the floor.

- Exhale and, while rolling through the spine, lift your rib cage off the floor to balance on your sit bones.

- Inhale and reach your arms toward your toes while maintaining a C curve in your back. Exhale and roll down the spine by articulating one vertebra at a time. Return to the starting position. Repeat for the desired repetitions.

Correct form
Keep your arms and legs straight throughout the movement.

Avoid
Avoid using a jerking motion as your raise or lower your arms and legs.

Annotation Key
Bold text indicates target muscles
Black text indicates other working muscles
* indicates deep muscles

transversus abdominis

iliopsoas*

pectineus*

adductor longus

sartorius

vastus medialis

triceps brachii

extensor digitorum

rectus abdominis

vastus lateralis

deltoideus posterior

vastus intermedius*

rectus femoris

tensor fasciae latae

441 Weighted Ball V-Up

Lie on your back with your legs extended and your arms raised overhead, grasping a weighted ball with both hands. Perform as you would a V-Up (#440). Repeat for the desired repetitions.

442 Single-Leg V-Up

Lie on your back with your arms extended over your head, hovering just above the mat behind you, palms up. Bend your knees and press them together. Anchor your feet into the floor. Extend one leg, straightening it from your hip and out through your foot. Raise your torso to form a 45-degree angle with the floor as you bring your arms up and over your head to reach forward toward your raised foot. With control, curl your spine down to the floor as you bring your arms up overhead and behind you again, keeping your knees pressed together. Repeat for the desired repetitions.

443 Balance Ball Jackknife Crunch

Sit on a balance ball trainer placed dome-side up on the floor. Raise your feet off the floor, bend your knees toward your chest, and extend your arms straight out at shoulder height parallel to the floor. Tighten your abdominals and straighten your legs until they are parallel to the floor. Bring your knees back toward your chest to return to the starting position, then continue for the desired repetitions.

444 Jackknife Crunch on Aerobic Step

Sit with your buttocks at the edge of an aerobic step or other elevated surface. Lean back slightly with your hands resting on the step, your fingers facing forward. Tighten your abdominals and straighten your legs until they are parallel to the floor. Bring your knees back toward your chest to return to the starting position, then continue for the desired repetitions.

445 V-Up with Swiss Ball Pass

Lie supine on the floor and extend your arms above your head. Bend your knees so that your feet are slightly off the floor and grasp a Swiss ball between your feet. Push your lower back into the floor, keeping your spine long. Contract your abdominals, and lift your upper back off the floor and forward, exhaling as you come up. Simultaneously reach upward with both arms and legs by folding your torso. Transfer the ball from your feet to your hands and return to the starting position. Repeat in the opposite direction to return the ball to your feet. Continue passing the ball from feet to hands for the desired time or repetitions.

446 Boat

Sit with your legs extended straight in front of you. Lean back slightly, bending your knees, and support yourself with your hands behind your hips. Your fingers should be pointing forward and your back should be straight. Exhale and lift your feet off the floor as you lean back from your shoulders. Find your balance point between your sit bones and your tailbone. Slowly straighten your legs in front of you so that they form a 45-degree angle with your torso. Point your toes. Lift your arms to your sides, parallel to the floor. Pull your abdominals in toward your spine as they work to keep your balance. Stretch your arms forward through your fingertips and elongate the back of your neck. Hold for up to 30 seconds and then release. Repeat for the desired repetitions.

447

Vertical Leg Crunch

When performing a Vertical Leg Crunch, you should feel a strong sense that your abs are not just getting stronger but also becoming streamlined and defined. With your legs up, your abdominals do almost all the work.

Annotation Key
Bold text indicates target muscles
Black text indicates other working muscles
* indicates deep muscles

transversus abdominis*

rectus abdominis

obliquus externus

rectus femoris

biceps femoris

vastus intermedius*

tensor fasciae latae

gluteus medius*

quadratus lumborum*

Correct form
Keep your arms and legs fully extended. Press your legs together, as if they were a single leg.

Avoid
Avoid jerking upward; use your lower-back muscles to drive and control the movement.

- Lie on your back with your arms extended behind your head and your legs extended in front of you, so that your body forms one straight line.

- Bring your arms over your head so they are reaching straight upward, your hands directly above your shoulders and your arms forming a 90-degree angle with the floor. Raise your legs until they are parallel to your arms.

- Using your abs to drive the movement, lift your shoulders off the floor, reaching your extended fingers towards your toes. Lower and repeat for the desired reps and sets.

448 Swiss Ball Vertical Leg Crunch

Grasping a Swiss ball between your feet, clasp your hands behind your head and perform a Vertical Leg Crunch (#447). Repeat for the desired repetitions.

449

Roll-Up

The Roll-Up is a classical Pilates mat exercise that will challenge your core muscles, flatten your abdominals, and strengthen your back. To execute this move properly, be sure to use the same control rolling down as you do rolling up.

- Lie on your back with your spine in neutral position and your ankles strongly flexed. Glide your shoulder blades down your back as you lift your arms over your head, extending them slightly above the mat behind you. Press your shoulders and your rib cage downward.

- Press your navel to your spine, and, in sequence, roll up each vertebra from the mat, reaching your arms forward into the space above your legs. It helps to really press your heels into the mat.

- Reverse the movement, rolling back down to the mat vertebra by vertebra, resisting the urge to lift your shoulders and collapse your chest. Continue for the desired time or repetitions.

deltoideus anterior

triceps brachii

extensor digitorum

rectus abdominis

transversus abdominis*

tibialis anterior

pectoralis major

serratus anterior

obliquus internus*

erector spinae*

obliquus externus

gluteus maximus

sartorius

rectus femoris

Correct form
Keep your abdominals and rib cage strongly engaged, and keep pressing your legs and heels into the floor for stabilization.

Avoid
Avoid using shoulder or arm momentum to roll up or down.

Annotation Key
Bold text indicates target muscles
Black text indicates other working muscles
* indicates deep muscles

450 Medicine Ball Roll-Up

Grasp a large Medicine ball and perform as you would the Roll-Up (#449). Keep your arms extended and the ball stable throughout the exercise. Repeat for the desired repetitions.

451 Roll-Up Triceps Lift

Lie on the floor with your spine in a neutral position. Hold a body bar in both hands. Bend your elbows so that your arms form a right angle with the body bar above your head. Keeping the rest of your body in place, straighten your arm muscles to smoothly roll up to a sitting position. Keep your arms extended with the body bar lifted overhead. Slowly roll back to lie in the starting position. Repeat for the desired repetitions.

452 Foam Roller Ab Pull-In

The Foam Roller Ab Pull-In is a multipurpose move that targets your abdominals while working your triceps. It also offers your hamstrings a massaging stretch and helps you improve your coordination and agility. Be mindful of how far you roll forward: the pull-in portion of the exercise is more challenging than the rolling forward.

· Sit on the floor with your legs outstretched in front of you, a foam roller placed under your knees. Plant your hands on the floor to support your torso, your fingers pointing toward your buttocks.

· Press into the floor to raise your hips, keeping your legs firm and your abdominals tight.

· Draw your hips backward through your arms, rolling your legs over the roller. Drop your head so that your gaze is directed at your thighs.

· Roll on the roller back to the starting position, keeping your hips lifted off the floor. Continue rolling forward and back for the desired repetitions.

453

Ab Roll-Out

The Ab Roll-Out is a challenging core-stabilizing exercise
from which many movements can be built. When you
correctly execute an Ab Roll-Out, you activate many
of the key core muscles. Recent studies have shown
that exercises such as this more efficiently activate
the rectus abdominis (the "six-pack muscle") and the
obliques than do Sit-Up or Crunch variations.

· Kneel on the floor with a foam roller placed
crosswise in front of you. Place your wrists on top
of the roller with your fingers facing away from you.

· Maintaining a neutral spine and making sure not to
sink your neck into your shoulders, roll forward on
your forearms.

· Continue to roll forward until the roller reaches
your elbows. Press into the roller, keeping your
hips aligned, then roll back to the starting position.
Continue rolling forward and back for the desired
time or repetitions.

serratus anterior

obliquus internus*

pectoralis major

obliquus externus

pectoralis minor*

quadratus lumborum*

triceps brachii

gluteus medius*

gluteus maximus

rectus abdominis

semitendinosus

transversus abdominis*

semimembranosus   biceps femoris

vastus lateralis   rectus femoris   tensor fasciae latae

Annotation Key
Bold text indicates target muscles
Black text indicates other working muscles
* indicates deep muscles

---

454 Ab Wheel

Kneel on the floor and grab the handles of an ab wheel,
then perform as you would the Ab Roll-Out (#453).

---

455 Swiss Ball Roll-Out

Kneel on the floor with your wrists resting on a Swiss
ball with your upper back straight and firmly supported,
your feet shoulder-width apart, your hips raised, and
your arms outstretched to your sides. Perform as you
would the Ab Roll-Out (#453).

456

Full-Body Roll

The Full-Body Roll stretches your glutes and tones your core muscles, especially the obliques. It is also a challenging range-of-motion exercise that demands impeccable form—you must move with control and precision.

· Lie with your legs outstretched and your arms extended out at shoulder height.

· Raise your right leg so that it is perpendicular to the floor. Turn your head to the right, and slowly rotate your lower body to the left, lowering your right leg until your foot is just above the floor.

· Roll back and lower your leg to the starting position. Continue to alternate sides for the desired repetitions.

Annotation Key
Bold text indicates target muscles
Black text indicates other working muscles
* indicates deep muscles

deltoideus medialis

deltoideus posterior

erector spinae*

transversus abdominis*

iliopsoas*

vastus intermedius*

rectus femoris

rectus abdominis

obliquus internus*

pectoralis major

semitendinosus

biceps femoris

pectoralis minor*

semimembranosus

deltoideus anterior

gluteus maximus

latissimus dorsi

gluteus medius*

obliquus externus

gluteus minimus*

457

Russian Twist

The Russian Twist works your abdominals and obliques with its torso-rotating motion. Regularly performing this exercise or its variations increases abdominal endurance and builds explosiveness in the upper torso, which may help boost your performance in sports such as swimming, baseball, hockey, golf, lacrosse, and boxing.

· Sit with your knees bent and your feet flat on the floor. Lift up through your torso. Raise your arms parallel to the floor so that your hands are outstretched above your knees.

· Rotate your upper body to the right, reaching toward the floor with your hands.

· Pass through the center and rotate to the left. Without stopping, continue moving with control from side to side at a steady pace for the desired time or repetitions.

Correct form
To keep your abdominals fully engaged, be sure to keep moving smoothly with control, without pausing between repetitions.

Avoid
Avoid holding your breath.

rectus abdominis

obliquus externus

vastus intermedius*

rectus femoris

latissimus dorsi

obliquus internus*

transversus abdominis*

iliopsoas*

tensor fasciae latae

vastus lateralis

458 Raised-Leg Russian Twist

Sit with your knees bent and your arms extended at shoulder height. Lift your feet off the floor and perform as you would a Russian Twist (#457). Without stopping, continue moving with control from side to side at a steady pace for the desired time or repetitions.

459 Seated Dumbbell Russian Twist

Holding a dumbbell in both hands, sit with your legs extended in front of you, knees bent and feet about hip-width apart. Lean back slightly and perform as you would a Russian Twist (#457). Without stopping, continue moving with control from side to side at a steady pace for the desired time or repetitions.

460 Medicine Ball Twist

Holding a Medicine in both hands, sit with your knees bent and your feet planted about hip-width apart. Lean back slightly and perform as you would a Russian Twist (#457). Without stopping, continue moving with control from side to side at a steady pace for the desired time or repetitions.

461 Tabletop Russian Twist

Sit with your legs elevated and your calves parallel to the floor. Lean back slightly and perform as you would a Russian Twist (#457). Without stopping, continue moving with control from side to side at a steady pace for the desired time or repetitions.

462 Spine Twist

Sit on the floor with your back straight. Extend your legs in front of you, slightly more than hip-width apart. Lift up and out of your hips as you pull in your lower abdominals. Twist from your waist to the left, then return to the center. Lift up and out of your hips again, twisting in the other direction. Return to the center and repeat for desired repetitions.

463 Oblique Roll-Down

Sit with your arms extended to the sides, parallel to the floor. Contract your abs and, while simultaneously rotating your torso to one side, roll backward. Rotate your torso back to the center. Rotate to the other side, return back to the center, and repeat the sequence for the desired repetitions.

464

Pull-Up

Often used in fitness qualifying tests, the Pull-Up is a fundamental upper-body-strength compound exercise that works a large number of muscles in your back, shoulders, and arms, with a particular emphasis on the latissimus dorsi. It calls for you to pull your own body weight, using an overhand, or pronated, grip. It is a versatile move that can be combined with other exercises to amp up the intensity—think Burpee with pull-ups, for example.

levator scapulae*

trapezius

rhomboideus*

teres major

brachialis

triceps brachii

latissimus dorsi

Correct form
Retract your shoulder blades to engage your back muscles; this tightens them so that you use your arm muscles less.

Avoid
Avoid arching or swinging; focus on keeping your body straight.

Annotation Key
Bold text indicates target muscles
Black text indicates other working muscles
* indicates deep muscles

· Using an overhand grip, place your hands just outside shoulder-width on a bar and hang until your arms are straight.

· Pull yourself up until your chest touches the bar, crossing your ankles if desired. Hold yourself in this position for one second and then lower yourself slowly to the hanging position. Repeat, performing the desired repetitions.

deltoideus anterior

pectoralis minor*

pectoralis major

biceps brachii

brachioradialis

extensor digitorum

465 Chin-Up

A Chin-Up reverses the grip that you use during a Pull-Up so that you grasp the bar in an underhand or supinated grip, with your hands about shoulder-width apart and your palms facing you. This places more focus on the biceps.

· Using an underhand grip, place your hands about shoulder-width on a bar and hang until your arms are straight. Bend your knees back and cross your ankles.

· Pull yourself up until your chin touches the bar. Hold yourself in this position for one second and then lower yourself slowly to the hanging position. Repeat for the desired repetitions.

466 Chin-Up with Hanging Leg Raise

Using an underhand grip, place your hands about shoulder-width or slightly wider on a bar and hang until your arms are straight. Bend your knees and cross your ankles. Perform as you would a Chin-Up (#465), but as you raise your chin to the bar, bend your knees, bringing them up toward your chest. Repeat for the desired repetitions.

467 Horizontal Strap Pull-Up

Loop a sturdy strap over the bar of a pull-up station. Lie down with your body perpendicular to the bar and grasp the ends of the strap. Using the bands, pull your body up toward the bar until your body forms a 45-degree angle from head to heels. Lower yourself slowly and repeat for the desired repetitions.

468 Body Row

Hang from a bar with your body in a flat plane. Move your feet away from the bar until your arms are straight, staying on your heels. Pull your body toward the bar until your chest touches it. Lower yourself slowly and repeat for the desired repetitions.

Pull-Up Grips

There are a wide variety of ways to perform Pull-Ups especially how you hold the bar. Here are some of the most common grip variations that you may encounter in your gym.

469 Wide Grip

Place your hands at least five inches (12.5 cm) wider than shoulder-width. This grip reduces the involvement of the pecs, which calls for you to work your back muscles more, especially the latissimus dorsi (more than the rhomboids).

470 Mountain Climber Grip

With the bar at your side, place one hand in front of the other, palms facing each other. Military trainees use this grip to simulate situations like pulling the body into windows or up ropes and climbing.

471 Close-Grip Underhand

Place your hands facing you at less than shoulder-width. Moving your hands closer together leads to greater pectoral activation.

472 Alternating Grip

Place one hand on the bar using an overhand grip and the other using an underhand grip at slightly wider than shoulder-width. This position improves grip strength, making it a great option for heavily weighted pull-ups.

473 Neutral Grip

Place your hands shoulder-width apart, palms facing each other, on a set of parallel handles. This grip places the least amount of stress on your shoulders, and it also emphasizes the brachialis, an upper-arm muscle.

474 Close-Grip Overhand

Place your hands facing out at less than shoulder-width. The narrow hand separation in this variation places emphasis on your lower lats.

475 Step Chin

Stand on a wall bar on one foot, grasping the top bar with an overhand grip. Extend your arms completely and bend the knee of your weight-bearing leg. Return by pulling your elbows down and pushing through the weight-bearing foot.

476 Dumbbell Step Chin

Stand on one foot on a lower bar of a wall bar, grasping the top pull-up bar with an overhand grip with one hand and holding a dumbbell in the other. Perform as you would a Step Chin (#475).

477 Vertical Rope with Alternate Grip

Place a flat bench under a gym rope. Grasp the rope with an alternating grip, one hand in front of your chin and the other slightly above your head. Step forward so that the rope hangs to one hip and place your heels on the bench. Pull down on the rope while simultaneously pushing down on your heels. Be sure to keep your knees bent and your torso upright throughout the movement.

478 Lateral Rope Pull

Place a flat bench under a gym rope. Stand on the bench and lean at a 30-degree angle from the floor, keeping your feet rigid and your weight on the edges of your shoes. With the rope at chest height, grasp it across your body with an alternating grip. Keeping the rope adjacent to your chest, move your arms downward and in toward your torso so that your knees extend slightly as your hips move upward.

479 Rope Chin

Stand on tiptoes with a gym rope directly in front of you. Grasp the rope with an alternating grip, one arm completely extended and the other slightly above your head. Step forward so that the rope runs down the middle of your body. Bend your knees slightly, and then hang on to the rope with just your hands. With both arms working evenly, pull down on the rope until your chin rises above your bottom hand.

480 Rope Chin with Hanging Leg Raise

Perform as you would a Rope Chin (#479), but at the start, bend your knees to 90 degrees. As you pull down on the rope, bring your knees toward your chest.

481

Deadlift

The Deadlift is a class bodybuilding power lift that is based on everyday movement. Just think of lifting a heavy object from the floor, hefting a laundry basket, or even picking up your toddler, and you know the mechanics of a Deadlift. You can perform it with just about any weight, from barbells to dumbbells to kettlebells to your own body weight. Its primary benefits are hip, leg, and lower-back strength, as well as improved position (posture) and range of motion (flexibility). Once you've mastered the basic version, try one of its many variations.

levator scapulae*

trapezius

rhomboideus*

erector spinae*

latissimus dorsi

gluteus maximus

obliquus internus*

obliquus externus

rectus abdominis

biceps femoris

adductor magnus

semitendinosus

semimembranosus

Correct form
To protect your lower back, contract your glutes and abdominals throughout the exercise.

Avoid
Avoid rounding your spine.

- Stand with your feet shoulder-width apart with a barbell at your feet. Lean over to grasp the weight with both hands.

- Using your core muscles as well as your arms, raise the barbell, hinging at the hips as you slowly rise to a standing position.

- Smoothly return the barbell to the floor, again hinging at the hips. Repeat for the desired reps.

482 Dumbbell Deadlift

Stand with your feet shoulder-width apart with a set of dumbbells at your feet. Lean over to grasp the weights and perform as you would a Deadlift (#481).

483 Single-Arm Dumbbell Deadlift

Stand with your feet shoulder-width apart with a dumbbell next to your right foot. Place your left hand behind your head and lean over to grasp the weight with your right hand. Perform as you would a Deadlift (#481).

484 Barbell Lever Sumo Deadlift

Wedge the end of a barbell into a corner. Get into a low Sumo Squat (#022) and grasp one end of the barbell. Stand up explosively and press the bar straight up.

485 Kettlebell Single-Arm Lift

Stand with your feet shoulder-width apart with a kettlebell between your feet. Lean over to grasp the weight with one hand and perform as you would a Deadlift (#481).

486 Single-Leg Straight-Leg Kettlebell Deadlift

Stand on your right leg and keep your left slightly behind your right heel, bearing little to no weight. Hold a kettlebell in your left hand. Bend your right leg very slightly as you bend over from your hip and lower the kettlebell toward the floor. Make sure that you keep your chest up and your back slightly arched. Your left leg remains in line with your spine throughout the exercise. Once you've touched the floor or gone as deep as you can, squeeze your glutes, hamstrings, and shoulder blades as you stand up on your right leg while your left leg returns to the starting position.

487 Sandbag Flip

Stand with your feet shoulder-width apart with a sandbag in front of you. Grasp the bag with your palms facing each another and squat deeply. Exhale and drive your torso upward and your hips up and forward. Push your feet into the floor, forcefully and quickly extending your knees and pulling upward on the bag with your upper back, shoulders, and elbows. Elevate onto your toes and follow through with your hands upward and forward away from your body, releasing the bag all in one fluid movement.

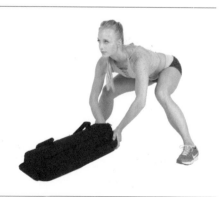

488

Bottoms-Up Kettlebell Clean

The Bottoms-Up Kettlebell Clean might look easy, but it really is a complicated move that takes your upper body through a range of movement that will help you burn fat and build muscle. It also helps you to develop hand strength and coordination.

- Stand upright with your feet shoulder-width apart, holding a kettlebell in your left hand. Swing the kettlebell backward, then bring it forward and above your head forcefully, squeezing the handle as you do so.

- Once your upper arm is parallel to the floor, hold the position, then lower your arm. Complete the desired repetitions, then repeat with the other arm.

palmaris longus
pronator teres
flexor digitorum
flexor carpi ulnaris

Annotation Key
Bold text indicates target muscles
Black text indicates other working muscles
* indicates deep muscles

Correct form
Keep your upper arm close to your body, as if you were tucking a purse or newspaper under your arm.

Avoid
Never use a weight heavier than you can safely control.

extensor digitorum
anconeus
triceps brachii
deltoideus anterior
deltoideus medialis
biceps brachii
pectoralis minor*
pectoralis major

489 Body-Weight Clean

Perform as you would the Bottoms-Up Kettlebell Clean (#488) without a kettlebell, instead making a tight fist. Be sure to contract your arm muscles throughout the exercise.

490 Kettlebell Swing

Stand over the kettlebell with your feet hip-width apart, chest up, and shoulders back and down. Squat down and grip the kettlebell with your palms facing you and your thumbs wrapped loosely around the handle. Stand tall, then, driving through your heels, explode through the hips to send the weight swinging upward from your quads, aiming to reach chest height with your arms extended. As the kettlebell begins to descend, shift your weight back into your heels while hinging at the hips and loading both the hamstrings and glutes. Receive the weight, allowing the kettlebell to ride back between your legs. As the weight makes the transition from backward to forward, drive through the heel to move into the next rep.

491 Kettlebell Overhead Arc

Being sure to use a weight you can safely control, perform a Kettlebell Swing (#490), bringing the weight above your head.

492 Kettlebell Row

Stand with your right leg extended in front of you. Keep your right leg bent and hold a kettlebell in your left hand. Rest your right hand above your knee and lean forward slightly. Bend your arm as you pull the weight up toward your chest. Lower and perform the desired repetitions, then repeat on the other side.

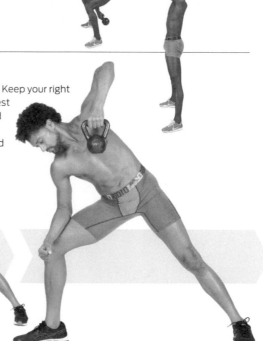

493

Double Kettlebell Snatch

The Double Kettlebell Snatch is an advanced bodybuilding move with multiple benefits: it builds strength, elevates heart rate, and increases mobility. Work with a trainer for the best results so that you learn proper lockout form and how to execute it to achieve your goals. Performing it quickly with lighter weights reaps maximum volume of oxygen benefits, while using heavier weights at low speeds results in full-body strength.

· Stand with your feet a little more than shoulder-width apart, holding a pair of kettlebells at your sides.

· Squat down, leaning forward slightly and sticking out your buttocks. Bring your arms between your legs so that the kettlebells are next to your inner thighs.

· In one swift, determined move, drive through your hips and swing the kettlebells overhead. Lower and repeat for the desired repetitions.

Correct form
As you swing the kettlebell upward, shrug your shoulders backward. This will pull the weights closer to your body, making them feel lighter when they reach the apex.

Avoid
Never use a weight heavier than you can safely control.

pronator teres
flexor carpi ulnaris
palmaris longus
triceps brachii
deltoideus posterior
biceps brachii
deltoideus medialis
pectoralis minor*
deltoideus anterior
pectoralis major
adductor longus
tensor fasciae latae
sartorius
iliopsoas*
vastus intermedius*
vastus lateralis
rectus femoris
adductor magnus
gracilis*
vastus medialis

Annotation Key
Bold text indicates target muscles
Black text indicates other working muscles
* indicates deep muscles

494 Clean and Press

Another classic bodybuilding power lift, the Clean and Press focuses on your shoulder muscles, but also works your trapezius, triceps, middle and lower back, abdominals, glutes, quadriceps, hamstrings, and calves, making it a highly effective full-body exercise. As well as building lean muscle, this challenging lift will also help you increase your endurance and stamina.

· Assume a high squatting position so that your upper legs are parallel with the floor. Hold a body bar in front of you with your arms straight.

· Using the muscles in your legs as well as your abdominals, rise to stand as you bend your arms to bring the bar to shoulder height. If you choose, extend one foot in front of the other.

· Move your feet to parallel position, hip-width or wider apart, and bring the body bar above your head. Hold for several seconds.

· Focus on breath and alignment as you bring the bar down to shoulder height in a controlled manner.

· Repeat the overhead lift and the controlled lowering for the desired repetitions.

495 Lateral Raise

Standing with your feet together, hold a dumbbell in each hand with your arms extended at your sides. Keeping your elbows and knees slightly bent, raise your arms out to your sides in wide arcs to about shoulder level. Slowly return to the starting position. Repeat for the desired repetitions. Lifting laterally activates your posterior deltoids and upper-back muscles.

496

4-Count Overhead

The 4-Count Overhead draws its inspiration from special forces stamina/endurance training exercises that call for teams to work in concert under a heavy weight. They must execute a variety of moves, including overhead presses, while instructors call the steps. Performed to a steady beat, the 4-Count Overhead simulates this kind of training while it works the muscles of your shoulders.

· Stand with your feet hip-width apart. With both hands, grasp a dumbbell of any weight that you can press overhead and bring it to your right shoulder. This is your starting position.

· Press the weight overhead with your arms straight for count 1.

· Lower the weight to your left shoulder for count 2.

· Press the weight overhead with your arms straight for count 3.

· Lower the weight to your right shoulder for count 4. Each time the weight touches your right shoulder equals one repetition.

Correct form
Move the weight around your head and not your head around the weight.

Avoid
Avoid arching your lower back.

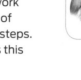

trapezius

rhomboideus*

Annotation Key
Bold text indicates target muscles
Black text indicates other working muscles
* indicates deep muscles

deltoideus anterior

deltoideus medialis

deltoideus posterior

497 Barbell Row

Stand with your toes pointing slightly outward, holding a barbell with both hands using an underhand grip. Keeping your lower back straight, bend your knees slightly and hinge forward at the hips. Lead with your elbows, pulling them toward the ceiling until the bar reaches the level of your upper waist. Return the bar to the floor so that your arms are fully extended and your shoulders are stretched downward. Repeat for the desired repetitions.

498 Upright Barbell Row

The upright row moves the target upward to the trapezius muscles of your upper back, neck, and shoulders and also works the deltoids and biceps. The narrower the grip, the greater the emphasis on the trapezius muscles. Stand upright grasping a barbell with a shoulder-width or slightly narrower overhand grip. With your elbows leading, pull the bar upward to neck height, allowing your wrists to flex as the bar rises. Lower the bar to the starting position, and then repeat for the desired repetitions.

499 Sandbag Slams

Place a sandbag at your feet, and then squat down to take a firm grip on the outside edges. Explode off your heels and drive the sandbag overhead while rising up onto your toes. Next, slam the sandbag onto the ground between your feet, snapping down onto your heels.

500

Shoulder Crusher

As its name implies, the Shoulder Crusher zeros in on your deltoids to give your shoulders a grueling, intense workout. Like many boot camp training exercises, it calls for you to perform a series of positions in rapid succession to the beat of a count. The counts can be called in any sequence, or you can perform the counts in the order listed below.

- Start with a dumbbell in each hand resting at the front of your thighs.

- Bring your hands to your chest for count 1.

- Move your arms straight out in front of your body at chest level for count 2.

- Keeping your arms straight, bring your hands overhead, and hold for count 3.

- Lower the weight to your shoulders, and hold for count 4.

- Press your arms overhead, and hold for count 5.

- Keeping your arms straight, bring them back out in front of your chest for count 6.

- Pull your hands into your chest for count 7.

- Drop your arms to the front of each thigh for count 8. Each time the weights hit your thighs equals one rep. Perform all steps for the desired time or repetitions.

deltoideus anterior

deltoideus medialis

deltoideus posterior

Correct form
When bringing the dumbbells overhead, make sure that your hands are directly above you and not in front of your center of gravity. Be sure to work with a weight that is not too heavy for your strength level.

Avoid
Avoid arching your lower back.

Annotation Key
Bold text indicates target muscles
Black text indicates other working muscles
* indicates deep muscles

501 Military Press

Stand holding a dumbbell in each hand and raise them to shoulder level with your palms facing out and your elbows bent. Press the weights up and toward each other as you straighten your arms, keeping a slight bend in your elbows at the top. Slowly bring down the weights and return to the starting position.

Index of Exercises

Credits

Photography

Naila Ruechel

Photography Assistant

Finn Moore

Models

Natasha Diamond-Walker
Abdiel Jacobson
Jessica Gambellur
Philip Chan
Anzie Dasabe
Lloyd Knight
Roya Carreras
Alex Geissbuhler
Daniel Wright

Additional Photography

Page 7 Kzenon/Shutterstock.com
Page 9 holbox/Shutterstock.com
Pages 12–13; 92–93 oneinchpunch/Shutterstock.com

Illustration

All anatomical illustrations by Hector Diaz/3DLabz Animation Limited

Full-body anatomy and Insets by Linda Bucklin/Shutterstock.com